Advanced Praise

"Diamandis' clear insights, combined with actionable strategies, will empower you to rewrite your own longevity story".

—**Tony Robbins**, Author, Coach, Business Strategist, author of the #1 *New York Times* bestseller, *Life Force*

"Diamandis delivers a clear and practical roadmap to unlock the secrets of a longer, healthier life. This book is a game-changer for anyone seeking to take control of their well-being and extend their years with vitality and purpose."

—**Mark Hyman, MD**, author of the #1 *New York Times* bestseller, *Young Forever*

"In LONGEVITY, Diamandis delivers a very clear and very actionable roadmap to maximize your healthspan, energy and vitality. A must-read playbook for those wanting to achieve Longevity Escape Velocity!"

—**Ray Kurzweil**, Inventor, Author and Futurist

"Peter's book LONGEVITY brilliantly distills the essence of lifelong health into tangible steps. This book is less a read and more an action plan, crafted to guide us all towards adding decades of health to our lives."

—**Anousheh Ansari**, CEO, XPRIZE, Astronaut

LONGEVITY

YOUR PRACTICAL PLAYBOOK
...on Sleep, Diet, Exercise, Mindset, Medications, and
Not Dying from Something Stupid

New York Times Bestselling Author
Peter Diamandis, MD

Chapter on Women's Health
By Helen Messier, PhD, MD

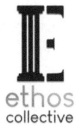

ethos
collective

Printed in the United States of America

Published by Ethos Collective™
PO Box 43, Powell, OH 43065
www.ethoscollective.vip

LCCN: 2023920647
Paperback ISBN: 978-1-63680-232-9
Hardcover ISBN: 978-1-63680-233-6
e-book ISBN: 978-1-63680-234-3

Available in paperback, hardcover, and e-book.
Cover photo credit: **Paul Smith**, @paulsmithphotography

This Longevity Practical Playbook includes many references. To access them, please scan the QR code below or visit Diamandis.com/Longevity-References.

Other Books by Peter H. Diamandis, MD

Abundance
Bold
Exponential Organizations 2.0
The Future Is Faster Than You Think
Life Force

Why I Wrote This Book

At the age of 62, I thankfully find myself in peak condition—physically, mentally, and energetically. A variety of performance and biomarker metrics bolster this sentiment. I've gotten here not by luck, but by effort and prioritizing healthspan. I'm on a personal mission to maintain my optimal health for the next decade, in order to intercept the next generation of therapeutics promising to decelerate, halt, and even reverse aging.

Over the past ten years, my primary focus has been the understanding and exploration of vitality and healthspan. I've immersed myself in research and devoured publications from the realm of biotechnology, healthspan, longevity, longevity diets, exercise strategies, sleep, and more. I've absorbed information from myriad podcasts, shared insights on my *Moonshots* podcast, and engaged in countless discussions at events like Abundance360 and Abundance Platinum. Additionally, my work with my own longevity-focused companies such as Fountain Life, Lifeforce, Celularity, Vaxxinity, and the $101M XPRIZE Healthspan have offered unique perspectives.

One thing for sure... there is a TON of information out there and it's hard to keep it all straight and accessible, which is why I wrote this book.

The aim of *LONGEVITY: Your Practical Playbook* is twofold: to simplify and to prescribe. I designed it to be digestible within a few hours and to serve as a practical reference guide you can turn to every day, or weekly as needed. A bridge to serve you over the next three to seven years leading up to the next wave of health breakthroughs.

Don't underestimate the value of this book due to its brevity. The challenge was not in accumulating material, but in curating it to be easily consumable, all while maintaining a rigorous backing of scientific research. After all, what's the point of amassing a library of health and diet books if they're left unread, or if you don't devise a clear, actionable plan for your wellbeing?

I sincerely hope you find this book beneficial, but more importantly, I hope it inspires you to prioritize your health. In today's world, health is indeed the new wealth. To quote one of my favorite sayings, "The individual who has health has a thousand dreams. The one without it has but one."

Here's to an extraordinary decade ahead.

Peter H. Diamandis, MD
Founder, Exec Chairman, XPRIZE Foundation
Exec. Founder, Singularity
Exec. Chairman, Fountain Life
Curator, Abundance360 & Abundance Platinum
Author: *Abundance, BOLD, Future is Faster, Life Force, Exponential Organizations 2.0*

"Life is short... Until you extend it!"

—Peter H. Diamandis, MD

DEDICATION

To my Abundance360, Abundance Platinum, XPRIZE, Singularity, and Fountain
Life Communities. All of you give me the gift of sharing my
passions and learnings with you.

Contents

"A key to longevity is having a future
that is bigger than your past."

—Dan Sullivan

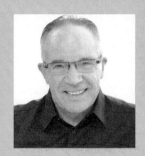

Introduction

We are in the midst of a healthspan revolution...

In this book, I'm sharing my own longevity practices—what I'm personally doing to extend my healthspan—which have been garnered from synthesizing well over three hundred interviews during my Abundance Platinum Longevity Trips, my *Moonshots* podcast, and in consultation with the medical team at Fountain Life.

In this first part of this book, we'll look briefly at the context in which this healthspan revolution is taking place and explore the concept of "longevity escape velocity."

Simply put, converging exponential technologies such as AI, genomics and other "omics technologies," CRISPR, gene therapy, cellular medicine, and invasive and non-invasive sensors are allowing us to understand why we age and how to slow, stop, and perhaps even *reverse* aging.

Experts predict that breakthroughs within the next ten years ***will enable us to add decades onto our healthspan.***

Healthspan refers to the period of life spent in good health, free from the chronic diseases and disabilities of aging. It emphasizes the quality of life lived rather than just the duration. In contrast, lifespan is the total duration of an individual's life, regardless of their health condition. While lifespan denotes the years lived, healthspan underscores the years lived healthily and actively.

Your mission is therefore to maximize your health and vitality by using the most advanced diagnostics to catch disease early, enabling you to stay healthy long enough to intercept the additional breakthroughs racing toward us.

Approaching Longevity Escape Velocity

So how long might we all live?

When I was in medical school in the late 1980s, I distinctly remember one Sunday afternoon watching a documentary on the topic of "long-lived sea life."

It turns out that bowhead whales from the Arctic can live for 200 years, and Greenland sharks double that life expectancy with an impressive lifespan of 400 and 500 years. These sharks can even have pups (babies) at 200 years old.

I remember thinking, "If they can live that long, why can't we?"

As an engineer, I figured it was either a hardware or software problem and it wouldn't be too long before we could solve it.

My dear friend Ray Kurzweil, Co-Founder of Singularity University and Futurist at Google, and Aubrey de Grey, a leading biomedical gerontologist, speak about a concept called "longevity escape velocity." It's an intriguing notion that goes something like this:

Today, by some estimates, science and medicine are adding about three months to your lifespan every year. In the near future (at some point), additional scientific breakthroughs will extend your lifespan *by more than a year* for every year you remain alive. Once that happens, we can begin to think about true longevity.

That concept is called longevity escape velocity.

I've asked many leaders in the health and longevity realm about their predictions. The answers vary widely, but there are two leaders in the field who give me the greatest confidence.

First is Ray Kurzweil, called "the restless genius" by *The Wall Street Journal* and "the ultimate thinking machine" by *Forbes*.

Kurzweil's written works became intellectual landmarks. His *New York Times* bestsellers *The Singularity Is Near* (2005) and *How To Create A Mind* (2012) became definitive texts in the field of artificial intelligence and exponential technologies. His next book, *The Singularity is Nearer*, is expected in mid-2024.

Beyond his brilliance, Kurzweil is most famous for his futuristic predictions.

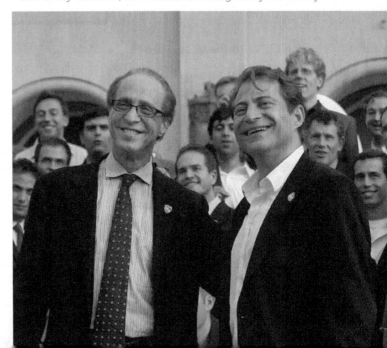

Peter & Ray Kurzweil, Co-Founders of Singularity University

To date, his written predictions, 147 in total, have demonstrated an astounding 86% accuracy (see his Wikipedia entry for more details on his predictions).

When asked about his prediction as to when we will reach longevity escape velocity, his answer was surprising and very encouraging, "For those in reasonably good shape, with reasonable means, I believe they will have access in the next 10 to 12 years."

Professor George Church of Harvard Medical School echoes a similar timeframe. George Church, PhD, is an indomitable figure at the forefront of genetics, synthetic biology, and longevity research, based at Harvard Medical School. His pioneering work transcends the conventional boundaries of science, having revolutionized genome sequencing, gene editing, gene synthesis, and the burgeoning field of age-related studies. He has founded over fifty cutting-edge synthetic biology companies that range from companies that are regrowing human organs to one (Colossal) that is bringing back extinct animals.

According to Dr. Church, "The exponential technologies that have improved the speed and cost of reading, writing, and editing of DNA and their resulting gene therapies now apply to the category of aging reversal."

He adds: "I think age-reversal advances could mean that we reach longevity escape velocity in a decade or two, within the range of the next one or two rounds of clinical trials."

So, what does that mean? Can we extend the healthy human lifespan past today's record of 122? Can humans live past 200 years? Or even indefinitely?

What if advancements in AI can significantly shorten the regular cycles of clinical trials? And what if we learn to prevent and eventually *eradicate* cancers, heart diseases, and Alzheimer's?

I recently sat down with Dr. David Sinclair, Professor of Genetics at Harvard Medical School and author of *Lifespan*, to discuss these topics for a recent episode of my *Moonshots* podcast.

I opened with a question about how long humans might be able to live: "Is there an upper age limit?" Sinclair's answer was inspiring: "There is no biological limit... of course there isn't," he began. "We are the same stuff as a whale that can live a lot longer than us (200 years), we're built of the same stuff as tortoises, pretty much the same stuff as trees that can live thousands of years, it's a software problem."

"I'm putting my career on the line," he continued. "It's a software problem and what's interesting about biology is that software encodes the ability to rebuild the hardware. So, we need to reset the software. When we do that in my lab, we find that tissues regenerate in animals; organoids, which are mini human organs, regenerate, they fix themselves and they function like they are new again. So it is, in my view, 99% a software problem."

Heredity vs. Lifestyle

How long you live is a function of many factors: where you were born, your genetics, your diet, and your mindset. Most people imagine that longevity is mostly inherited, that the genetic cards you are dealt have predetermined your lifespan.

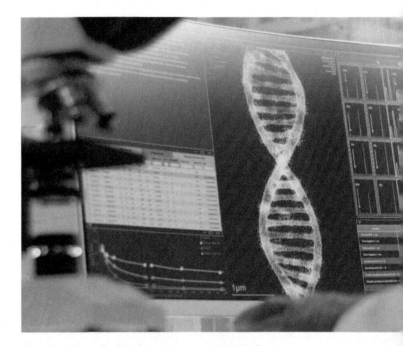

Heredity has a limited impact on your longevity

You may be surprised by the truth.

In 2018, after the analysis of a 54-million-person ancestry database, scientists announced that lifespan has little to do with genes.

In fact, **heritability is accountable for roughly 7% of your longevity**.

The highest estimates for heritability verge around 30%—which still means at a minimum, you're 70% in control of how you age.

The power of shaping your healthspan is much more in your hands than you might have imagined.

Closing Thoughts

It is this idea of extended healthspan that is my motivation for putting together this practical playbook on longevity. It is also my desire to create something that is simple and easy to reference and consume. My own experience is that many longevity "how to" books are way too long, include too much theory, and are impractical to consume and use.

I would like to thank Helen Messier, PhD/MD, Chief Medical and Chief Scientific Officer of Fountain Life for her review and support in creating these protocols and for her addition of an important chapter on women's health. Many thanks as well to George Shapiro, MD, Medical Innovation Officer of Fountain Life, for his input on therapeutics.

In the short chapters that follow, I share details on what I've learned, synthesized, and adapted—the practical playbook I currently use in my effort to extend my healthspan.

"I implore you to consider adopting some of these and to think through what YOU would do with an additional 30 years of healthy life..."

—Peter H. Diamandis, MD (October 2023)

Peter's Legal Disclosure

I am an educator, entrepreneur, and scientist. ***I am not a clinician and cannot make clinical recommendations for the prevention or treatment of any disease. In making these suggestions, I am expressing only my own views and sharing what I am personally doing for my health.***

No one should start taking any supplement or medications without first checking with his or her personal physician. Some supplements can be dangerous for people with certain pre-existing medical conditions, and supplements can interfere with some prescription drugs. Supplements can and will affect people differently.

In general, the FDA is limited to post-market enforcement because, unlike drugs that must be proven safe and effective for their intended use before marketing, there are no provisions in the law for the FDA to approve dietary supplements for safety before they reach the consumer. **Note**: The evidence of benefit for most of these supplements comes from laboratory experiments and/or from epidemiology data, not from human clinical trials.

Supplements should only be purchased from trusted retailers and brands. Testing has shown that many supplements are tainted with unlisted ingredients and/or do not contain the amount of the supplement listed on their label.

For additional, more detailed recommendations in the categories of sleep, exercise, diet and supplements, please read *Life Force*, a book jointly written by me in partnership with Tony Robbins and Robert Hariri, MD, PhD.

Chapter One:
Peter's Longevity Diet

"100 to 120 years is a nice range, but what I want is to live with passion and aliveness. I want energy, vitality and the strength during that time. I want to be able to keep rejuvenating. That to me matters the most."

—Tony Robbins

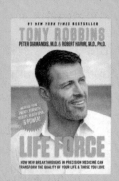

You Very Literally Are What You Eat.

The nutrients (or non-nutrients) you consume become your body and mind. Do you overindulge in good-tasting (sugar-rich) but destructive foods? Or do you craft a sensible diet and practice intermittent fasting to maximize your energy and longevity?

There are actions you can take right now to increase your potential healthspan, and ensuring that you have a healthy diet that works for you is an easy place to start.

In this chapter, I'll discuss a few simple steps you can take to improve your diet based on my discussions with Dr. Mark Hyman, Dr. Helen Messier, and Dr. Guillermo Rodriguez Navarrete. Below, I'll also share details on what I eat (and don't eat) to maximize my healthspan.

My Longevity Diet

What you eat and drink, how much you eat, when you eat, and especially how you eat and drink are critically important.

The problem is that there is no "one diet" that serves everyone. In fact, thousands of different diet books have been published, and over 5 million are sold in the U.S. alone every year, so the field is diverse and complicated at best.

The following is what I personally do. I do believe that some of the details below are

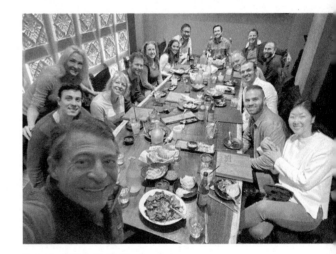

Peter and his PHD Ventures team

somewhat fundamental for everyone. Ultimately, what is best for you will depend upon your genetics, age, microbiome, environmental exposures, health objectives and your physician's advice. (**Note**: Additional details and backup information for many of these practices can be found in my book, *Life Force*.)

Below is a summary related to the diet practices that I follow:

What I Do **NOT** Eat

No Added Sugar or High Glycemic Foods: I think of **sugar as a poison**. I do my best to stay away from sugar, simple carbohydrates, and processed starches. The human body never evolved to consume the levels of sugar in most diets today. Human physiology evolved on a diet containing very little added sugar and virtually no refined carbohydrates. In fact, refined sugar probably entered into our diets by accident. It is likely that sugarcane was primarily a "fodder" crop used to fatten pigs, though humans may have chewed on the stalks from time to time.

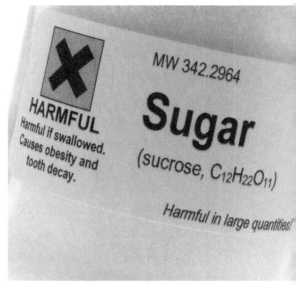

Sugar is a poison

The effects of added sugar intake can be devastating, including higher blood pressure, inflammation (cardiac and neuro), weight gain, diabetes, fatty liver disease, and fuel for cancer. Increased blood sugar levels are directly linked to an increased risk for heart attack and stroke. On the other hand, reduced blood sugar levels have been linked to lower blood pressure and cholesterol and have been shown to lower the risk of heart attack, stroke, and heart-related death.

Sugar is addictive and hard to quit. Studies with rats have shown that sugar can be as addictive as cocaine. Every year as part of **Abundance360**, I join nutritionist Dr. Guillermo Rodriguez Navarrete (Fellow of the American College of Nutrition, FACN, and a member of the American Society for Nutrition) to take members through a **"22-day No-Sugar Challenge."** We do this as a group on WhatsApp. The communal nature of "doing it together" is incredibly useful. It takes about three weeks for your brain and body to eliminate cravings for sweets and begin craving healthier foods that satisfy more of your actual nutritional needs. The good news is that you can break the addiction, and the results can be monumental.

In my recent discussions with Mark Hyman, MD, a physician and author of the bestselling book *Young Forever*, he notes, "When you eat sugar, it slows your metabolism down, and it increases hunger hormones. So, you're hungrier, you're gaining weight, and you can't burn the fat." Sugar consumption increases levels of the hormone insulin, which has the primary purpose of turning that sugar into stored fat.

Sugar intake results in significant hormonal problems—and perhaps most shockingly, new evidence proves that sugar shrinks your brain's hippocampus, which is your memory center, leading to poor memory and reduced overall brain volume. So, the next time you have a sugar craving, think about how it may literally shrink your brain cells.

As Dr. Hyman remarks, "93% of Americans are metabolically unhealthy... they have high blood sugar, high cholesterol, high blood pressure, or they're overweight, or they have already had a heart attack or a stroke." This means, in effect, that a mere 6% of us are in good metabolic health. "And," Dr. Hyman continues, "that's driven by our diet primarily."

Personally, I don't eat dessert. When it's offered at the dinner table or restaurant, I have conditioned myself to say "no" immediately (before the plate ever hits the table), so I'm not tempted to even have it on the table in front of me. When I'm feeling a craving for something sweet (and everyone does), on occasion, I will satisfy it with a bit of dark chocolate (>75% dark cacao).

What Else I DON'T Eat: Beyond avoiding sugar, simple carbohydrates, and processed starches, which all turn readily into sugar in your body, **I don't eat dairy products or beef**. My food allergy testing indicates that I have an immune response to the casein protein component in dairy that can drive inflammation. I avoid beef because of its high saturated fat content and the association of red meat with cancer, especially colon cancer as well as cardiovascular disease. Although grass-fed beef can be a healthy part of some diets, it is easier for me to decrease consumption by avoiding it altogether.

What I DO Eat

A Whole-Plant Diet, as much as I can. There's no question that consuming whole plants is a major plus. As such, I'm focused on spinach, broccoli, Brussels sprouts, avocado, asparagus, and most other unprocessed veggies with a heavy helping of extra virgin olive oil. I'll typically have a Greek salad with added avocado and protein such as fish, chicken, or legumes for lunch.

Vegetables are key to a healthy diet

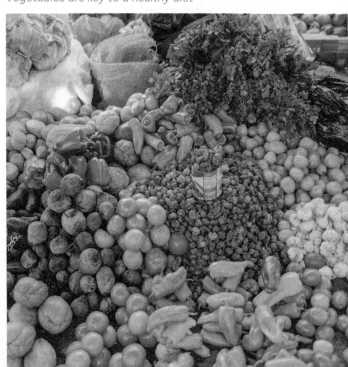

As Dr. Helen Messier says, "**Eat the rainbow**" (and that doesn't mean Skittles or Fruit Loops). Eating a wide variety of colored fruits, vegetables, and spices corresponds to the consumption of different phytochemicals, vitamins, minerals, and antioxidants, each with unique health benefits. For example, plants contain thousands of natural chemicals called "phytonutrients" or "phytochemicals." Many of these are responsible for the color of the plants. These chemicals have protective properties that can benefit human health when consumed. In addition, different colors often indicate different antioxidants. Antioxidants are compounds that help protect our bodies from damage by free radicals, which can contribute to chronic diseases and aging. When I see different colored vegetables on the table, I do my best to eat them all!

Slow Down / Breathe Deep / Vitamin "O": Have you ever heard of vitamin O (oxygen)? This is another important concept that Dr. Messier has shared with me—it's all about breathing deep to activate your parasympathetic system. If you're eating "on the run" or in front of your computer or (worst of all) in front of the TV watching CNN, this is the worst way to digest your food.

To maximize both enjoyment and the healthy absorption of nutrients and full digestion of your meal, it's all about activating your parasympathetic system. To do this, take a few deep breaths to slow down your heart rate, increase your oxygen intake, and increase your parasympathetic system while having dinner. This is why people say grace or share what they are grateful for at the beginning of a meal. Activating your parasympathetics will increase HCl production in your stomach in order to digest the food. People should eat in a mindful fashion.

Nuts, Beans & Legumes for Protein: I try and take in as much plant protein as possible from nuts (typically macadamias, walnuts, and almonds), as well as properly soaked and prepared beans and legumes which are high in protein: soybeans, lentils, white beans, cranberry beans, split peas, pinto beans, kidney beans, black beans, navy beans, and lima beans (see below).

Nuts are a great source of protein

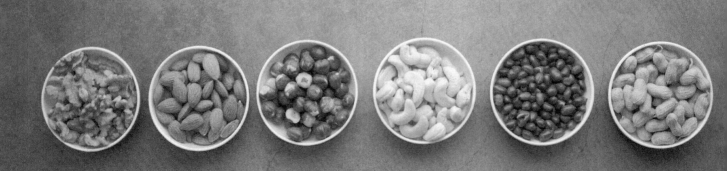

Protein: Protein is an essential building block of life. You need it for building and repairing tissues like muscles, bones, and skin, as well as for producing hormones and enzymes, transporting nutrients and oxygen, supporting immune function, and providing energy to each of your cells.

In my podcast with Dr. Hyman, he noted: "Some believe we should limit protein (especially animal protein) and amino acids to silence mTOR and activate autophagy." But, he adds, the data isn't so clear: when we abstain from animal proteins altogether, and the longevity pathway mTOR becomes "silenced for long periods, we can't create new proteins or build muscle." For maximum longevity, we need to balance the anabolic mTOR pathway, which builds up our tissues with the catabolic AMPK pathway, which stimulates autophagy and cleans up all the damaged cells and proteins.

Typically, I eat protein from the following sources:

- Fish (salmon) 3 times per week, eggs, and chicken (I avoid tuna, swordfish, and large fish like the plague because they are high in mercury and getting worse every single year!).
- Whey protein shakes 3 times per week (especially on days I'm lifting weights).
- **Nutri11** protein drink (served hot) is my coffee replacement each morning. With zero sugar and 11 grams of protein, I LOVE the taste (sweetened by monk fruit).
- Plant protein shakes on all other days. In particular, I love **Ka'Chava** (chocolate), which I enjoy as a breakfast and sometimes as a snack.
- Lentils, about 18 grams of protein per cooked cup (240 ml).
- Chickpeas, as well as black, kidney, and pinto beans, are substantial sources of protein, offering around 15 grams per cooked cup (240 ml).
- Quinoa and Amaranth contain all nine essential amino acids. A cup of cooked quinoa or amaranth has about 8 – 9 grams of protein.
- Green Peas: One cup (160g) of cooked green peas contains 9 grams of protein.
- Almonds, sunflower seeds, flaxseeds, and chia seeds are all good protein sources.

Protein Intake Goals: This year, I am endeavoring to add 10 pounds of additional muscle mass to my frame, and to accomplish this, I need to take in a lot of extra protein. Typical advice suggests 0.80 grams of protein per pound of body weight (1.6 grams per kg). But what I've read suggests that is too low, especially as we need to maintain muscle mass as we get older, so my personal goal is now 1.0 gram of protein per pound of body weight. I take in a whopping 150 grams per day (I weigh about 145 pounds).

NOTE: It is important not to consume a day's worth of protein all in one sitting but instead to spread it out over three to four servings during the course of the day. Doing this will maximize muscle protein synthesis, enhance recovery, sustain an anabolic state, optimize nutrient utilization, and also manage appetite.

During my days when I'm doing a heavy-weight workout and trying to consume maximum protein, here's an example of what I'll consume:

Item:	Grams Protein	Calories:
Whey protein shake	25 grams	120
Almond milk	2 grams	80
Nutri11 drink	11 grams	145
Blueberries	--	40
Athletic greens	2 grams	50
Chicken breast	43 grams	230
Broccoli	3 grams	30
Whey protein shake	25 grams	120
Almond milk	2 grams	80
Chicken breast	43 grams	230
TOTAL	156 grams	1,125

*Note: As noted above, I recently discovered a great "hot" protein drink that I have used to replace my coffee in the morning called **Nutri11**, produced by nutritionist Dr. Guillermo Rodriguez Navarrete. Nutri11 has zero sugar and 11 grams of protein. I LOVE the way it tastes.*

What I Do NOT Drink

Sodas: I've eliminated 100% of sodas from my diet, given the added sugar and phosphoric acid.

Fruit Juice: I've eliminated 100% of high-fructose fruit juices, which can spike my blood sugar. Fructose, especially in liquid form, can increase uric acid levels, blood pressure, and appetite.

Alcohol: I've eliminated almost all alcohol, save for an occasional glass of red wine. Alcohol truly has very few medicinal benefits, is a major driver of microbiome disruption and leaky gut, and can play havoc with sleep. While about 20% of adult Americans use alcohol to help them fall asleep, new research shows that while alcohol may bring on sleepiness, it can disrupt sleep and, over time, cause insomnia by interfering with the body's system for regulating sleep.

What I DO Drink

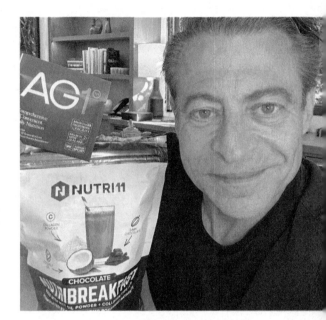

Water + Athletic Greens: I aim to drink 2+ liters of water per day, prioritizing fresh spring water like Fiji. In the morning, occasionally, I'll mix in a package of **Athletic Greens (AG1)**. AG1 is a low-calorie (50 calories in total), nutrient-dense, comprehensive daily drink packed with 75 vitamins, minerals, and whole food-sourced ingredients. It supports key areas of health, including energy, immunity, gut health, and hormonal balance. Its all-in-one formulation is designed to boost overall wellness, making it a healthy addition to your daily routine.

Peter drinks AG1 & Nutri11 every day

Morning Hot Drink Routine: I will typically have a morning cup of decaf coffee. I recently learned from my genetics (from my Fountain Life whole genome testing) that too much caffeine isn't the best thing for me. As an alternative to coffee, I will typically have a hot mug of **MUD\WTR**, which is a black tea powder containing a number of beneficial mushrooms, or a hot mug of **Nutri11** (high in protein with no sugar or carbs). On the tea side, I personally love Moroccan mint tea (with a touch of pure honey).

Coffee: When I was going through medical school, I probably would average six or more cups of coffee per day, always black without cream or sugar. I just wanted the caffeine kick. Recently when I checked my genetics at Fountain Life, I found out that I'm a slow metabolizer of caffeine, and getting more than a cup per day could actually be bad for my health. So, I've effectively stopped (and it was easier than I thought). I haven't cut it out completely, but I've switched almost exclusively to decaf.

Fasting / Timing of Meals / Calories

Fasting / Timing of Meals: Over the years, I have experimented with various time-restricted or "intermittent fasting" diet programs. In years past, I would fast for 19 hours per day, having dinner at 6 pm, skipping breakfast, and eating lunch around 1 pm. Last year, I gave up this practice for two reasons: first, there seems to be no real benefits. A 2020 clinical trial of 116 volunteers on a sixteen-hour (off), eight-hour (on) eating regimen found no weight loss and no cardiometabolic benefits (see Peter Attia's' book *Outlive* for details). The second reason for giving up on intermittent fasting is because of my desire to consume 150 grams of protein over the course of the day on a distributed basis. I focus on whole foods, and along with the protein mentioned above, this keeps me feeling full; thus, my overall calorie intake is well controlled. Minimizing overall calories has proven to promote longevity in almost all animal models tested, including non-human primates.

ProLon Fasting Mimicking Diet: There does appear to be good evidence that multi-day fasting periods are pro-longevity-supporting autophagy. But let's face it, doing a water fast for 5 days is really, really, really hard!

One of the best ways to get the benefit of longer fasts without the pain is something called the **ProLon Fasting Mimicking Diet**, which is a guided, shake-based fast that supports healthy weight loss and cellular rejuvenation. It's a 5-day program that is relatively painless and something I've been doing twice per year. My Longevity physician tells me that, ideally, I should do this once a month for 3 months in a row. More information is available here www.prolonfast.com.

CGM – Measuring My Blood Glucose: High blood glucose levels are a challenge to the body. High blood glucose is a major cause of inflammation in the body and a contributor to heart disease and dementia. I use a "continuous glucose monitor (CGM)" such as those supplied by **LEVELs** as well as the **FreeStyle Libre-3.** My goal is to measure which foods spike my blood glucose. It also keeps me aware of my eating habits in the same way that my OURA ring helps me monitor my sleeping habits. Stress, lack of sleep, and timing of eating can all impact your blood sugar response even to the same food.

FreeStyle Libre 3

GLUCOSE IN RANGE

98 → mg/dL

Peter uses a CGM to monitor blood glucose

Freestyle Libre-3 readout: No spike between 6am – 8am with Nutri-11 and Whey Protein shake. Spike between 8am – 9am due to weight workout.

Meal Sequencing – The Order in Which You Eat Your Food Matters (A LOT):
Picture this: You're seated at your dinner table, a colorful plate of food before you, and you're about to take the first bite. What if I told you that the order in which you eat your meal could have a significant impact on your health, specifically in managing blood sugar levels and supporting weight control? Welcome to the world of meal sequencing, a concept that modern dietetic sciences have unveiled as a powerful tool in the quest for better nutrition.

Imagine your plate divided into three parts: carbohydrates, protein, and vegetables (fiber). Now, let's rearrange them in a way that can transform your eating experience and its effects on your body.

First in Line – Fiber-Packed Vegetables: Begin your culinary journey with the vibrant, fiber-filled bounty of non-starchy vegetables. Think kale, broccoli, bell peppers, and spinach. The more colorful, the better. Starting with vegetables serves two important purposes. First, it kickstarts your meal with a burst of nutrients and hydration, making you feel more satisfied from the get-go. Second, the fiber in vegetables helps slow down the digestion of other foods to come. This means you won't experience those rapid spikes in blood sugar levels that can lead to energy crashes and unwanted cravings.

Next Up – Protein Power: After your veggies, protein takes center stage in stabilizing your blood sugar levels and curbing your appetite. Enjoy a succulent piece of grilled chicken, fish, or a hearty serving of plant-based tofu or legumes. Protein-rich foods provide a sense of fullness and satisfaction that helps you control portion sizes. Plus, they work in harmony with the fiber from your vegetables to create a dynamic duo for regulating blood sugar.

Last but Not Least – Carbohydrates: Finally, if you opt to eat carbohydrates, do that last. Eating your carbohydrates last allows your body to prioritize the digestion of fiber and protein, reducing the potential for blood sugar spikes.

"Let your food be your medicine and your medicine be your food."

— Hippocrates

Chapter Two:
Peter's Exercise Practice

"Extending the healthy human lifespan will increase global abundance and uplift humanity. The equation is simple; longer healthier lives means more time spent at our productive best which means more innovation."

—Peter H. Diamandis, MD

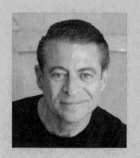

Exercise Is The Single Most Important Pro-Longevity Activity You Can Undertake.

If you are over 60 years old, exercising just twice per week with weights (resistance) doing push-pull type exercises (push-ups, pull-ups, deep knee bends, etc.) has the effect of reducing all-cause mortality by 50% and reducing your risk of cancer three-fold.

So, what type of exercise should you strive to incorporate in your life? How often and how much?

When I think of exercise, I'm using it to accomplish two objectives: My first goal is to increase muscle mass, and my second goal is to optimize my metabolic and mitochondrial health.

Below, we'll dive into both of these. I'll share my exercise routines, and explain why exercise is so important as a pro-longevity practice.

Increasing Muscle Mass

Adding muscle to your frame is fundamental for health and longevity. As I mentioned earlier, my personal goal for the year ahead is to add 10 additional pounds of skeletal muscle.

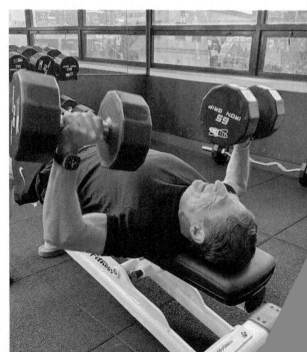

Peter does a heavy weight workout 3 times per week

Why? A number of studies have demonstrated a direct correlation between longevity and muscle mass. One study published in the journal *Aging* looked at data from over 10,000 people and found that those with the highest muscle mass were 30% less likely to die during the study period than those with the lowest muscle mass. Another study published in *The Lancet Diabetes & Endocrinology* found that people with sarcopenia (a condition characterized by low muscle mass) had a *50% increased risk of death from all causes.*

One reason for the benefit of increased muscle mass is its role in preventing injuries from falling. As it turns out, many deaths occur when prolonged sarcopenia (i.e., loss of muscle mass) ultimately leads to a fall, resulting in a fractured hip or pelvis, followed by hospitalization, pneumonia, and, ultimately, death. (**Note:** According to a 2019 study in *Acta Orthopaedica*, in adults over the age of 65, the one-year mortality rate after a hip fracture is 21% for those whose fracture is surgically repaired. If the fracture is not repaired, the one-year mortality jumps to 70%.)

For this reason, building and maintaining muscle mass is absolutely critical, and this is not a "once and done" activity. Building muscle needs to become part of your regular routine. Muscle mass decreases approximately 3 - 8% per decade after age 30, and this rate of decline is even higher after age 60.

There are a number of things that we can do to help preserve muscle mass, including exercising regularly with heavy weights, eating a healthy diet high in protein, getting enough sleep, and managing stress.

What I Do to Build Muscle

Heavy Weight Workout: I work out three times per week using heavy weights for both my upper and lower body (Sundays at Gold's Gym with my trainer TR and twice per week with Speck at Equinox). Each session is an hour long, guided by a trainer who pushes me harder than I can typically push myself. If I can occasionally squeeze in a fourth workout during the week, I will absolutely prioritize that. The only real challenge is travel, and the way that I try to overcome my excuses during travel is to work out with my Strikeforce team member, Dr. Yianni Psaltis, who normally travels with me.

Tonal Workout: This year, in my pursuit of adding muscle mass, I invested in an at-home all-in-one AI-enabled workout system called Tonal, which I make an effort to use on those days when I'm not lifting free weights. The Tonal system strives to marry the best of strength training with the innovation of smart technology.

At its core, Tonal is a wall-mounted unit that harnesses electromagnetic resistance to simulate weights, allowing users to engage in a wide variety of strength training exercises without traditional bulky gym equipment. Accompanied by an interactive display, the system intelligently adapts to each individual's needs, calibrating workouts in real time and providing expert coaching through guided routines.

The importance of the Tonal system lies not just in its space-saving design but in its ability to deliver personalized, efficient, and dynamic workouts. It redefines the boundaries of traditional training by offering a tailored experience that can accelerate muscle growth, enhance strength, and revolutionize the way we understand home fitness.

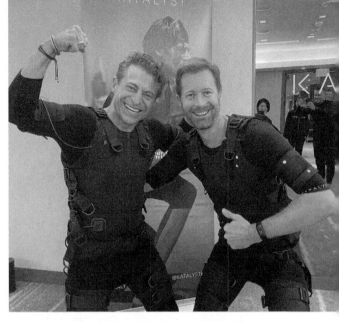

Peter uses a Katalyst suit for brief workouts to maintain muscle mass

Katalyst Workout: Last year, I purchased a **Katalyst Suit** for use at home. Katalyst uses electricity to stimulate your muscles to contract, called electro muscle stimulation (EMS). This is a way to help you build strength or power in a 20-minute, at-home session. This helps me maintain muscle mass when I'm short on time and it also helps me create variety in my workout. One recommendation is that you *remain very well hydrated* when using the Katalyst Suit and don't overdo it.

Creatine: Before each heavy weight workout, I consume 5 grams of creatine. Research shows supplementing with creatine can double your strength and lean muscle gains compared to training alone. Creatine, a natural substance in muscle cells, enhances muscle growth and strength in several ways: by increasing ATP production for high-intensity workouts, promoting cell signaling for muscle repair, boosting cell hydration for muscle size, stimulating protein synthesis, reducing protein breakdown, and lowering myostatin levels to increase muscle growth potential.

At-Home Quick Workouts: In between my heavy weights, I will work out at home with simple exercises: push-ups, abdominal bicycle, sit-ups, v-ups, squats, and lunges. One of the great apps I love for pushing me through a daily exercise routine is called the **7-Minute Workout**. It's developed by Johnson & Johnson and is free in the App Store. The app includes a high-intensity, circuit training workout, with aerobic and resistance exercises using only body weight.

Measuring Muscle Mass / Whole-Body Composition: Measuring how your muscle mass changes is important. You must measure what matters. To do this, I use the **InBody H20N**, a smart weight analyzer that goes beyond weight, measuring whole-body composition including lean muscle and body fat percentage. It helps me monitor and gamify my goals. I also measure my body composition in greater detail during my annual upload at Fountain Life. DEXA scans and MRI measurements give enhanced detail of my lean and fat tissue and where it is located.

VO2 Max & Mitochondrial Health

Having plenty of muscle is great, but what about the metabolic health of your muscle and its mitochondria? In other words, what is the ability of your mitochondria (the powerplants of your cells) to convert oxygen and glucose or fat into energy for your body in an efficient fashion? VO2 max, or maximal oxygen uptake, is the way that we measure that efficiency. It's a measure of the maximum amount of oxygen that an individual can use during intense exercise and a key indicator of cardiovascular fitness and aerobic endurance. A higher VO2 max generally indicates a greater capacity for aerobic exercise and endurance.

VO2 max is important for several reasons, including:

- Cardiovascular health, reducing the risk of heart disease and stroke;
- Physical fitness and mobility;
- Chronic disease prevention, reducing the risk of diabetes, hypertension, and certain types of cancer;
- Mental health and cognitive function, reducing the risk of depression, anxiety, and cognitive decline, including conditions like Alzheimer's disease; and
- Longevity.

Several studies have found a direct correlation between VO2 max and longevity. Higher VO2 max levels in middle age have been associated with increased survival rates in older age. "The relationship between VO2 max and all-cause mortality is quite good," says Dr. Michael Joyner, an anesthesiologist and fitness expert at the Mayo Clinic. "The odds of dying in the next 10 years are markedly low if your VO2 max is high."

How I Work on Improving My VO2 Max

1. Steady-State Cardio: I endeavor to get at least 3 (ideally 4) days each week of moderate "Zone 2" cardio exercise for 45 – 60 minutes. Zone 2 training has been shown to be the best way to improve the functioning and efficiency of your mitochondria. For me, this involves getting my heart rate to 110 bpm – 115 bpm and holding it steady through light jogging / brisk walking, cycling, or tennis. My go-to is a stationary bicycle where I can take my board and team Zoom calls that otherwise would have me sitting around.

Here's how you calculate your **Zone 2 heart rate**:

- **First, calculate your maximum heart rate ("max HR"),** which is equal to 220 minus your age. For me: 220 − 62 = 158
- **Second, calculate the lower limit of Zone 2,** which is equal to your max HR x 60%. For me: ~100 bpm
- **Third, calculate the upper limit of Zone 2,** which is equal to max HR x 70%. For me: ~110 bpm

It's worth noting that you can also do a lactate threshold test that will determine your exact Zone 2 heart rate, which is something I do at Fountain Life during my annual upload. This involves getting on a stationary bike, peddling at increasing speeds, and having a medical technician sample your blood lactate levels from a finger prick at regular intervals.

2. Interval Training Cardio: Beyond Zone 2 training 1 or 2 days a week, I replace a steady-state cardio workout with a High Intensity Interval Training (HIIT) workout. I warm up for 5 – 10 minutes then alternate between 1 minute of high-intensity exercise (such as sprinting or fast cycling) and 1 – 2 minutes of low-intensity recovery. I repeat this cycle for 20 – 30 minutes.

Walking or Tennis Meetings: During and after the COVID-19 pandemic, I've made it a habit to do many of my in-person meetings as "walk and talk" sessions. My daily goal is to exceed 10,000 steps measured on my Apple Watch / iPhone. I wear a heart rate monitor that allows me to get my heart rate into Zone 2 (which, for me, is about 110 bpm) and maintain it there for an hour, 3 times per week (i.e., my Zone 2 training). Recently, I've added the idea of a tennis meeting, having a conversation while hitting the ball around for an hour on the court.

Walking Desk/Stationary Bike: To help me reach and exceed my 10,000-steps goal, I have been using a **LifeSpan walking desk** whenever I've been office-bound. Every Zoom or phone call can be done on a walking desk. As I've been saying for years, "Sitting is the new smoking!" In addition, I recently purchased a **Technogym stationary bike** that helps me track my Zone 2 heart rate and delivers a double duty benefit for every Zoom board call.

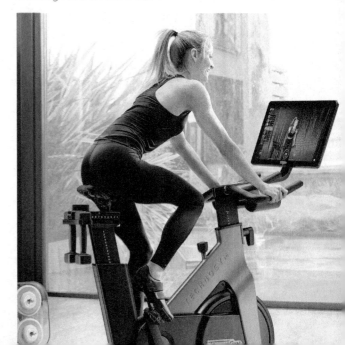

Peter uses a Technogym stationary bike for cardio & tracking Zone 2 heart rate

Measuring Cardio / Heart Rate: I use a Polar Verity Sense to measure my heart rate during workouts. I wear an optical heart rate monitor on my forearm, providing freedom of movement and multiple options for viewing and recording my workouts.

Avoiding Injury

As we grow older, our biggest enemy is no longer sugar or even lack of sleep; **it's INJURY**. An injury can cause a sequence of events that can unravel all of the pro-longevity work you've done. A fall that breaks any bone or tears a ligament can result in a prolonged period of bedrest that can wipe away many months of muscle accumulation or VO2 max improvements.

The antidote here is a set of protocols focused on balance and flexibility/stretching. As we get older, we tend to get stiffer and more unstable. Maintaining or gaining flexibility and working on proprioception, which is an awareness of the position and movement of your body, is critical in preventing injury. Personally, I must admit that flexibility is my Achilles' heel, and I probably need to sign up for some yoga classes.

A Regenerative Medicine Story: At this point, I'll tell a short story regarding injury and regenerative medicine. About twelve years ago, I required a rotator cuff repair of my right shoulder. Recovery was slow and painful. Three years ago, while gardening, I tripped on a tree root, landed on my left shoulder, and again required a rotator cuff repair. Because on this occasion I had access to exosomes, after surgery I injected exosomes into the repair site 3 times during the first month. While this is simply my personal observation, I'm clear that the recovery of my left shoulder was substantially faster and less painful. I'm looking forward to the research studies that are forthcoming this decade to demonstrate the power of exosomes and stem cells in muscular-skeletal reconstructions.

Stretching helps you avoid injury

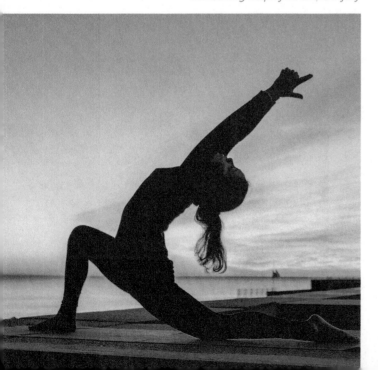

Why Exercise Matters So Much

In a 2018 study published in *The Lancet*, researchers looked at the link between physical activity and mortality.

With data from over *1 million people*, the study found that individuals who engaged in 150 minutes of moderate-intensity exercise per week had a *28% lower risk of death from any cause*.

But the data gets even more compelling.

Subjects who engaged in 750 minutes per week—or 12.5 hours—had a mind-blowing **42% lower risk of death** compared to those who never exercised.

There is no known therapy or drug with this type of well-studied effect on human lifespan.

Even just regular, frequent movement—especially outside, in fresh air—has the potential to transform your mood, maintain your heart health (protecting you from the number one killer in the world!), and significantly boost your creativity and problem-solving skills. That's because when you exercise, your muscles release myokines into your bloodstream. These myokines go to your brain, where they regulate physiological and metabolic responses as well as affect cognition, mood, and emotions. They also aid in the formation of new neurons and increased brain plasticity.

Another recent study found that participants who walked over 4,000 steps a day had healthier brain tissue, better memory, as well as superior cognitive function compared to those who walked fewer than 4,000 steps per day.

So, if you don't yet exercise regularly, start somewhere. Ideally, you'll get to 10,000 steps a day plus 3 times a week of weight training. But as you can see, just 4,000 steps a day can be the difference between life and death, between a healthy brain and Alzheimer's, or a number of other debilitating diseases.

A Benchmark to Follow Your Progress – A Target to Shoot For!

In 2022, a friend, Regan Archibald, collaborated with my coach, Dan Sullivan, Founder of Strategic Coach®, to create "Your Fitness 50 Benchmark" as a simple means of self-assessment, goal setting, and tracking progress.

> "Living to 100 isn't the problem most of us will face, the problem is the condition in which we arrive."

As Archibald and Sullivan have said, living to 100 isn't the problem most of us will face, the problem is the condition in which we will arrive. Imagine having the fitness levels of the healthiest 50-year-olds at the age of 100. Your future self will appreciate the time you spend taking care of your health, and the Fitness 50 Benchmarks are a simplified way to increase longevity.

Each of the Fitness 50 Benchmarks can be viewed as a diagnostic predictor of diseases caused by aging and serve as an early indicator for all-cause mortality. I think that Sullivan's Fitness 50 Benchmarks are the easiest way to measure your progress toward your life extension goals. No blood draws, stool tests, or DNA swabs are needed.

Your Fitness 50 Benchmarks

Successfully go to Fit to Fitter to Fittest in each category

FIT		FITTER		FITTEST	
Push Ups: 50 Seconds	15	Push Ups: 50 Seconds	25	Push Ups: 50 Seconds	40
Plank Hold	1 Minute	Plank Hold	2 Minute	Plank Hold	3 Minute
Grip Test: Dead hang	30 Seconds	Grip Test: Dead hang	60 Seconds	Grip Test: Dead hang	90 Seconds
Squats: 50 Seconds	20	Squats: 50 Seconds	35	Squats: 50 Seconds	50
Wall Squat Hold	30 Seconds	Wall Squat Hold	60 Seconds	Wall Squat Hold	90 Seconds
Lunges: 50 Seconds	20	Lunges: 50 Seconds	35	Lunges: 50 Seconds	50
Sit-To-Stand: 50 Seconds	6	Sit-To-Stand: 50 Seconds	8	Sit-To-Stand: 50 Seconds	10
Sit-To-Rise: No Hands	2	Sit-To-Rise: No Hands	1	Sit-To-Rise: No Hands	0
Single Leg Balance: 50 Seconds	20	Single Leg Balance: 50 Seconds	35	Single Leg Balance: 50 Seconds	50
1-Mile Walk/Run/Elliptical	12 Minutes	1-Mile Walk/Run/Elliptical	10 Minutes	1-Mile Walk/Run/Elliptical	8 Minutes
25 Burpees	4 Minutes	25 Burpees	3 Minutes	25 Burpees	2 Minutes
ACHIEVED		**ACHIEVED**		**ACHIEVED**	

Dan Sullivan and Regan Archibald Lifetime Extender Collaboration © eastwesthealth2022

The 3 levels are Fit, Fitter, and Fittest. I see them as motivation to make improvements no matter what age or fitness level you are at. I like to work on each of the 11 benchmarks simultaneously once a week, but you could choose to perform some of the benchmarks in groups or test them as a single activity. The purpose is to have a baseline fitness threshold that you can enjoy when you are 100 years old.

Below are my June 2023 numbers and a simple chart I will use to follow my progress over the years ahead.

Peter's Fitness 50 Benchmark Numbers

	Reference Fittest	Peter's June '23	Peter's June '24	Peter's June '25
Push Ups: 50 Seconds	40	**90**	_____	_____
Plank Hold:	3 Min	**3 Min**	_____	_____
Grip Tests: Dead hang	90 Sec	**135 Sec**	_____	_____
Squats: 50 second	50	**50**	_____	_____
Wall Squat Hold:	90 Sec	**180 Sec**	_____	_____
Lunges: 50 Seconds	50	**41**	_____	_____
Sit-To-Stand: 50 Seconds	10	**13**	_____	_____
Sit-to-Rise: No Hands	0	**0**	_____	_____
Single Leg Balance: 50 Secs	50 Sec	**>120 Sec**	_____	_____
1-Mile Walk/Run/Elliptical	8 Min	**10 Min**	_____	_____
25 Burpees	2 Min	**1.5 Min**	_____	_____

An Explanation of Each Category

Push-ups: Being able to perform 40 push-ups (modifications are fine) can reduce stroke and heart disease by 96%, increase strength, and improve growth hormone. *Cardiovascular Health and Strength.

Plank Hold: Improves posture, strengthens the core, and increases flexibility and endurance. Planks increase the basal metabolic rate, decrease the fat percentage, and have been shown to improve immunocyte counts. *Metabolism, Flexibility, Strength, Endurance, and Immune Function.

Grip Strength: Increases in strength reduce blood pressure and risk of stroke. It improves testosterone and growth hormone, signals muscle readiness for the entire body through the brain, and can be a stand-in measurement for full body strength and muscle mass. *Cardiovascular Health and Strength.

Wall Squat Hold: Enhances lower body stability and strength while reducing resting blood pressure and improving lumbar stability. *Balance, Alignment, Cardiovascular Health, Strength.

Lunges: Benefits the posterior muscles (hamstrings, glutes, and lower back) better than other movements. Corrects instability and improves balance. *Strength, Balance, and Alignment.

Sit-to-Stand: Core strength, endurance, and balance and is a predictor of mortality. *Strength, Balance, Endurance.

Sit-to-Rise: Musculoskeletal fitness predictor for longevity, balance, and coordination. *Strength, Balance, and Coordination.

Single Leg Balance: Decreases the chances of strokes and improves cerebral circulation and vascular health. Promotes flexibility and prevents cognitive decline while warding off premature mortality. *Flexibility, Balance, and Cardiovascular Health.

1-Mile Run/Elliptical/Rowing/Swimming: Improves cardiovascular function, decreases chances of stroke, improves endurance and strength. Increases cognitive function and fitness. Rowing, swimming, and the elliptical are just examples of alternatives to running. Feel free to test yourself on any endurance-related activity for 8 – 12 minutes to see how you fare. *Endurance, Cardiovascular Fitness, and Brain Health.

Burpees: Increase blood flow, lowers blood pressure, and improves strength, coordination, and endurance. Stimulates fat burning and metabolism and lowers the risk of all-cause mortality. *Endurance, Fitness, Strength, and Cardiovascular Health.

"...participants who walked over 4,000 steps a day had healthier brain tissue, better memory, as well as superior cognitive function, compared to those who walked fewer..."

Chapter Three:
Peter's Sleep Practices

"*Sleep is Mother Nature's best effort yet to counter death.*"

—Matthew Walker, PhD

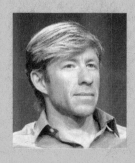

You need 7 to 8 hours of sleep each night.

Getting enough sleep is one of the most underappreciated and most important elements of extending your healthspan. If you think you're one of those people who can get away with 5 or 6 hours of sleep, the scientific evidence is not on your side.

Sleep expert Dr. Matthew Walker, author of the excellent book *Why We Sleep*, says that sleep is the single most effective thing we can do to reset our mental and physical health each day.

As Dr. Walker told me during my Abundance Platinum Longevity Trip, "Sleep is Mother Nature's best effort yet at immortality."

There is a direct relationship between how well you sleep and how long you live.

In this chapter, I'll discuss the power of sleep and what I'm doing to improve my sleep and increase my longevity.

The Power of Sleep

In *Why We Sleep*, Dr. Walker points out that *close to 0%* of the total population can get away with less than 6 hours of sleep a night without harming their health.

For most people, regularly getting 8 hours of sleep boosts memory retention, enhances concentration, augments creativity, stabilizes emotions, strengthens the immune system, enhances athletic performance, and staves off deadly ailments like cancers and heart disease.

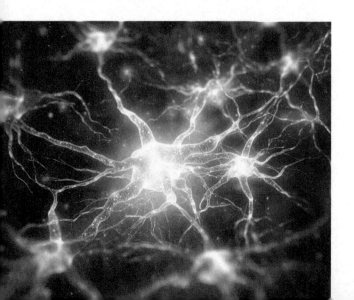

Still not convinced?

For the human brain, the difference between regularly getting a good night's sleep and a bad sleep is a decrease from *100% to 60%* in the brain's ability to retain new facts. Or, as Dr. Walker puts it, a sliding scale between "acing an exam and failing it miserably."

Good sleep boosts brain performance

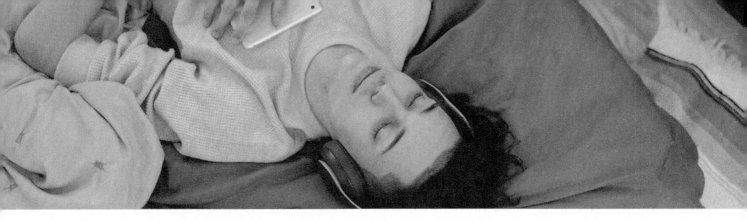

Listening to an audiobook or music helps to wind down before sleep

Sleep plays a critical role in learning and memory. Throughout the night, we fluctuate between rapid eye movement (REM) sleep, where dreaming occurs, and deeper non-rapid eye movement (NREM) cycles. These cycles are responsible for transferring the information accumulated throughout the day from short-term memory to long-term memory.

REM sleep and the mental images created during it also help fuel our creativity by generating new connections between ideas that may not be obvious while we're awake. Dr. Walker's research has shown that REM sleep acts like *overnight therapy* by allowing us to process difficult experiences with rehearsed ease.

Sleep gives our bodies a vital opportunity to recover from the stresses of the day. It aids recovery from inflammation, gives our cells a chance to restock their energy stores, and stimulates muscle repair. It is during sleep that the glymphatic system in our brains clean out all the accumulated junk helping to prevent neurodegenerative diseases and keeping our brains working optimally.

Regularly failing to complete our sleep cycles leads to significant drops in the time taken to reach physical exhaustion, reduced muscle strength, faster build-up of lactic acid, and lower blood oxygen.

Need more evidence? Every spring when we move the clocks forward one hour (Day-Light Savings Time), and we all lose an hour of sleep, hospitals report a 24% spike in heart-attack visits around the US. Just a coincidence? Probably not. "That's how fragile and susceptible your body is to even just one hour of lost sleep," says Dr. Walker. "Daylight saving time is a kind of global experiment we perform twice a year," he continues, "and the results show just how sensitive our bodies are to the whims of changing schedules."

With that in mind, here's what I'm doing to ensure I consistently get a good night's sleep.

My Sleep Practices

Forty years ago (during college and medical school), I would pride myself on making do with as little sleep as possible. My target was typically 5.5 hours. My usual excuse was, "I'll have plenty of time to sleep when I'm dead." I would routinely take red-eye flights so I could sleep on the flight and hit the ground running. ***Boy was I wrong. I wish I knew then what I know now!***

I now prioritize getting 8 hours of high-quality restful sleep, and here's how I do it. (Much of this information is available in more detail in the books *Life Force* and *Why We Sleep*.)

How Long and When: Today, my absolute target is 8 hours of sleep, with 7 hours as a minimum. It doesn't mean I always achieve that, but I always try. While I used to be a night owl, staying up routinely until 2 am, over the past decade I've shifted my sleep schedule to a much earlier bedtime. I'm usually in bed by 9:30 pm and asleep by 10 pm, and typically wake on my own around 5:30 am to 6 am.

Wind Down & Bedtime: One of the most important keys to getting a good night's sleep is consistency in your bedtime, complemented by a consistent "wind-down" period.

Standard Bedtime: This is <u>more important than you might expect</u>. Setting and sticking to a routine is critical for high-quality sleep. Eight hours of sleep between 10 pm and 6 am is *not* the same as 8 hours between 12 am and 8 am.

Wind-Down Period: For me, this is 30 – 60 minutes, typically between 8:30 pm and 9:30 pm, when I turn down the lights, wear my blue-light-blocking glasses, and slow down my routine. No TV. No Computer. I'll get into bed and either meditate on the day (focusing on what I'm most grateful for) or listen to a book on Audible (typically science fiction).

Peter's Sleeping Kit: Manta Sleep Mask, mandibular device, blue-light-block glasses & Oura Ring

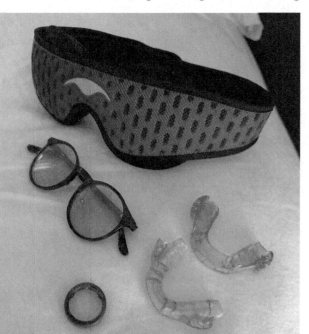

Eye Mask: I use a **Manta Sleep Mask** (MantaSleep.com), which I love. It's super comfortable, blocks out all light, and avoids putting pressure directly on your eyes. I've become addicted to my Manta mask and own 3 of them, and I always travel with one wherever I go.

Staying Cool at Night: A cooler room supports quality sleep by aiding the body's natural sleep-friendly drop in core temperature. It also reduces the likelihood of disruptions like sweating and restlessness. This contributes to maintaining uninterrupted, deep REM sleep, and promoting overall sleep quality and health. In my routine, there are two things I do in this area:

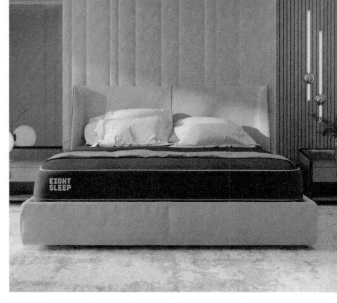

Eight Sleep cooling mattress pad

- **Room Temperature:** First off, I follow Dr. Walker's advice and set my room temperature air conditioning at a chilly ~64 degrees F (18.2 degrees C). This helps me get my core body temperature down to enter deep sleep.

- **Cooling Mattress Pad:** Second, I purchased **Eight Sleep**, a system that covers the mattress (under the bedding) and cools you down to a chosen temperature. I typically set this at "-5 degrees." The nice thing about the Eight Sleep mattress is that you can dial a temperature curve through the night. Meaning that in the middle of the night, the system can automatically get cooler, and in the morning, I have it warm up (I set it at +4 degrees).

Blue-Light-Blocking Glasses: Our brains evolved in the savannas of Africa to wake up with the sunrise and sleep when the sun sets. Bright blue light, which you'll get from an early sunrise, or your computer screen, is a signal to your brain to wake up. Red light, similar to the spectrum of a sunset, is a signal for you to release melatonin and prepare for sleep. In our normal high-tech world, bright lights, computers, cell phones, and TVs just before bed are sleep disruptors. Putting on a pair of blue-light-blocking glasses can help prevent giving your brain the wrong signals.

Given this knowledge, around the time of sunset (usually as much as 2 hours before going to sleep), I'll endeavor to put on a pair of blue-light-blocking glasses to ensure my body produces optimal melatonin levels to help me fall asleep more quickly and stay asleep throughout the night. On the other side of sleep, I love to get outside to see the sunrise, to give my visual system and brain the signals to wake up and enter my day fully powered up.

Mandibular Adjustment Device: Sleep apnea sucks. It's a sleep disorder characterized by repeated interruptions in breathing during the night, leading to fragmented sleep and decreased oxygen intake. Over time, untreated sleep apnea can contribute to daytime fatigue, impaired cognitive function, mood disturbances, and an increased risk of accidents. Furthermore, it is associated with hypertension, heart disease, stroke, and type 2 diabetes.

In the past, I used a CPAP (continuous positive airway pressure) machine, which works, but they are clumsy, uncomfortable, and look more like a torture device. Now, I use a specially fitted upper and lower mouth guard called a "mandibular advancement device." This device is a dental appliance used in the treatment of sleep apnea and snoring. It is designed to help keep the airway open during sleep by repositioning the lower jaw (mandible) and tongue slightly forward. Plus, it also prevents me from grinding my teeth. I love it so much that I can't go to sleep without it. There's no single brand I can recommend. Ultimately, to get one, visit your dentist to get an impression taken and get it fitted.

Evening Entertainment: One change I've made that makes a huge difference is eliminating TV in bed before sleep, plus staying off my phone and computer for the last 30 minutes before sleep. Instead, what I love doing is using Audible to listen to a book and set the timer for 15 or 20 minutes. I guess that's the adult equivalent of being read a bedtime story!

Lifeforce Peak Rest sleep supplement

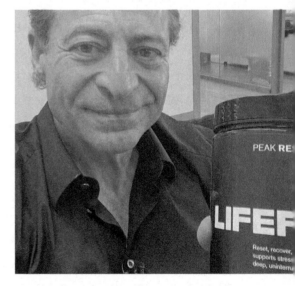

Sleep Supplement: So what do I do when I have jetlag, or am having trouble getting to sleep? One product I use is **Peak Rest by Lifeforce**, which includes a slow-release melatonin formulation, magnesium glycinate, L-Glycine, L-Theanine, and vitamin A. A second hack for me is to have a pad of paper and pen next to my bed to write down my ideas when my brain is over-active in the middle of the night. Getting it out of my head and onto paper allows me to relax and get back to sleep.

Oura Ring – Measuring My Sleep: While the Oura ring isn't a magical device that will put me to sleep, it does allow me to gamify my sleep by giving me a detailed numeric evaluation of how well I slept through the night.

Each morning, one of the first things I do is look at my daily "Readiness Score" and "Sleep Score" (see details at the end of this chapter). My goal is to always get at least a score of 90 on each metric (which I don't always achieve, but it's my target). Many times, just the thought that I will be measured in the morning is motivation enough to get to sleep early and minimize any alcohol or late-night food intake.

No Late-Night Eating: One important recommendation for getting a great night's sleep is to avoid having any food within 2 hours of going to sleep (so, typically 7:30 pm for my desired 9:30 pm bedtime). This gives my body enough time to begin digestion and prevent a full stomach that can lead to heartburn. Not eating before bed also promotes autophagy, which is the way your body cleans out all the misfolded proteins and cellular debris. Your microbiome is also much healthier when you don't eat right before bed since it allows the beneficial organisms that do best in a calorie-poor environment to thrive.

No Caffeine After Noon: Caffeine has a half-life of 4 to 6 hours in individuals who are fast caffeine metabolizers and 8 to 10 hours in slow caffeine metabolizers. This means it takes that amount of time for the quantity of caffeine in your body to be reduced by half. Since I am a slow caffeine metabolizer (which I know from my Fountain Life genetic analysis), I have chosen to drastically reduce and almost eliminate my caffeinated coffee consumption. On occasion, I may have half a cup when I wake up, but then I will switch to decaffeinated.

Why Sleep Matters

According to a study in Rand Health Quarterly, poor-quality sleep costs the US over $400 billion per year in lost productivity.

The same study estimates that more than half a million days of full-time work are lost every year due to people sleeping less than 6 hours.

On an individual level, for most people, sleep is often the first thing they give up. But the popular belief that "you can sleep when you're dead" is fundamentally damaging to your health, happiness, and longevity.

For example, regularly getting less than 6 or 7 hours of sleep each night doubles your risk of cancer and can increase the likelihood that you'll develop Alzheimer's disease. Insufficient sleep can also contribute to major psychiatric conditions such as anxiety and depression.

One of the key lessons from *Why We Sleep* is: **If humans had been able to evolve with the ability to get along with less sleep, then we would have.** Yet evolutionarily, our bodies retained the need for 8 hours.

PLEASE make getting a solid 8 hours of sleep a priority for yourself.

My Oura Ring Sleep Readouts

If you use an OURA ring, this type of readout (Sleep and Readiness Scores) on your smartphone will look familiar. My typical OURA Score will range between 88 and 97 (97 is my all-time high). My goal every night is to get a sleep score >90. I provide these below as a reference. Note that in a healthy sleep structure, the majority of your deep sleep should take place in the first half of your night and REM sleep in the second half.

The Oura Ring tracks 20+ biometrics

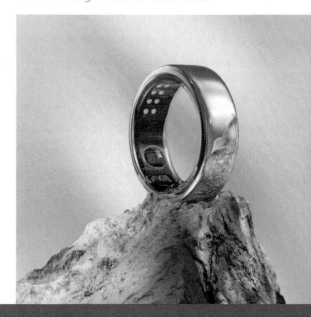

"Human beings are the only species that deliberately deprive themselves of sleep for no apparent gain. Many people walk through their lives in an under slept state, not realizing it."

—Matthew Walker, PhD

Oura Sleep Score

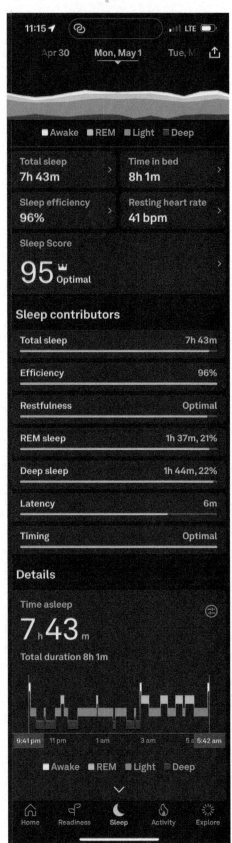

Peter uses the Oura Ring to gamify his sleep

Oura Readiness Score

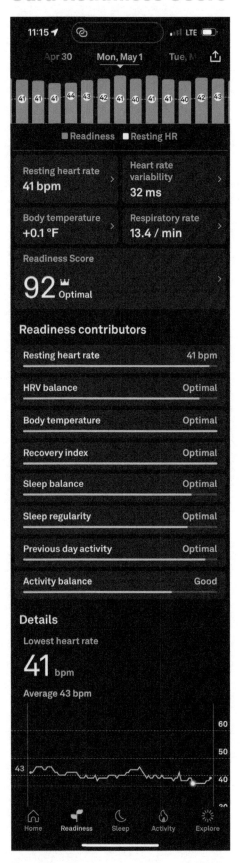

Peter aims to get at least 90 on his Sleep and Readiness scores

Chapter Four:
Peter's Annual Fountain Life Upload

(i.e., Not dying from something stupid)

*"Our aim should be to help our patients
die young as late as possible."*

—Tenley Albright, MD

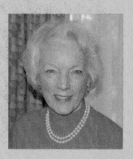

Reality: Your Body is Masterful at Hiding Disease

Most of us have *no idea* what's really going on in our bodies. We're all optimists, thinking we're fine and everything is in great working order. But as it turns out, your body can be quite masterful at hiding the early and middle stages of disease. What do I mean? Consider the following:

- 70% of all heart attacks have no precedent. No pain, no shortness of breath, and, in many instances, nothing on a typical coronary CT. Many times, the first symptom of cardiac disease will be a heart attack (which can sometimes times be fatal). Coronary heart disease affects about 18.2 million Americans age 20 and older, killing nearly 366,000 annually.

- 70% of all cancers that are fatal turn out to be the result of cancers that are not routinely tested for by today's medical system (for example, pancreatic cancer as opposed to prostate and breast cancer, which are tested for routinely).

- Someone with Parkinson's doesn't develop tremors until nearly 70% of the Substantia Nigra neurons are gone.

- Most individuals have no symptoms from a growing cancer until it has reached stage 3 or stage 4, at which point the chances of a full remission are greatly reduced.

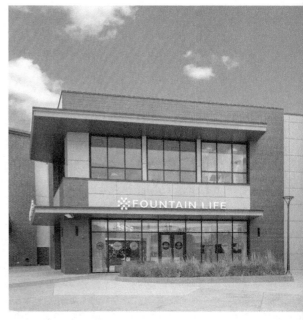

Fountain Life has multiple locations in the US and is expanding internationally

Perhaps you've known a friend or colleague who died in their sleep or someone who went to the hospital with some type of pain only to find out that they had some advanced stage of disease. **Here's the issue:** Whatever disease was discovered during that hospital visit didn't just start that morning. It's probably been going on for some time, months if not years, they just had no idea because they hadn't bothered to look. Most of us know very little about the inner workings of our bodies—we know more about what's going on in our car or refrigerator!

But as it turns out, you can know with great confidence if you have a cancer, aneurysm, or metabolic disease. Today advanced diagnostics are able to evaluate your health on a regular basis, with the goal of finding disease at the earliest stage possible.

This is why I co-founded Fountain Life with Tony Robbins and Dr. William Kapp (and now serve as Executive Chairman). Fountain Life is a global platform that provides advanced diagnostics and vetted therapeutics to promote a longer, healthier, and more vital life.

In this chapter, I'll discuss the Fountain Life platform and how I use it to increase my longevity and avoid dying from something stupid, as well as using it to vet the most advanced and effective therapeutic treatments available.

My Annual Fountain Life Upload

Every year, I go through a **Fountain Life "upload"** as part of their **APEX Membership** program (there are also other levels, including a Digital Membership, SNAP, and EDGE).

The APEX diagnostic program gathers more than 150GB of data about you to determine whether you currently have, *or are at risk for developing,* any of the leading causes of a shortened health and lifespan, specifically cardiovascular disease, cancer, aneurysms, metabolic disease, and neurocognitive dysfunction.

Should any dysfunction be discovered, a Functional Medicine-trained team will employ a systems-based approach to uncover the molecular drivers and provide an ongoing plan to restore cellular health.

The APEX Membership is designed for individuals who desire access to the most advanced comprehensive testing and access to a Functional Medicine-trained longevity physician able to interpret your results and implement a roadmap based on your advanced testing.

Fountain Life offers preventative, predictive & personalized care

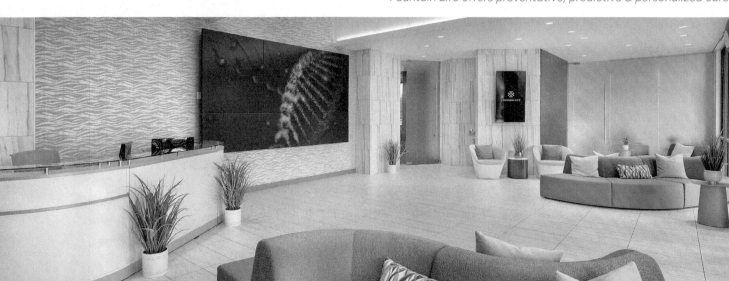

APEX Member Diagnostic Testing

The following are the major imaging and blood biomarker tests that are conducted as part of this membership offering:

- \>100 Clinical Biomarkers
- Brain MRI & Full Body MRI
- AI-enabled Coronary CT Angiogram (looks for vulnerable soft plaque)
- Blood-based Multi-Cancer Early Detection Testing
- DEXA Scan
- Metabolic Testing
- Whole Genome Sequencing
- Mouth & Gut Microbiome Analysis
- Retinal Scan
- Low-dose Lung CT
- Nutritional Testing
- Toxin Testing
- Strength Testing
- Sleep Apnea Testing
- Epigenetic Testing (identifies biological age.)

A detailed listing of what's included in a Fountain upload follows.

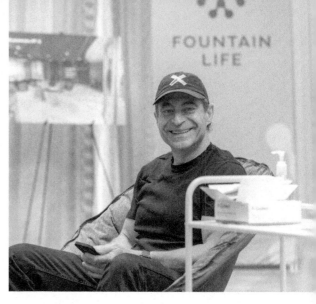

Peter gets his annual Upload at Fountain Life

Why Should You Look?

As mentioned above, the body is amazing at compensating for any disease, thereby masking its impact. Add to that fact that we are all optimists about our health. We think we're doing fine until that moment when you're rushed to the hospital.

The numbers tell the story.

Out of 100 seemingly healthy adults who go through a Fountain Life screening, 2.0% have a cancer they didn't know about, 2.5% have an aneurysm, and 14.4% of seemingly healthy members have a serious life-threatening finding they need to address.

Some people say, "I really don't want to know." My response is: "You are definitely going to find out if something is wrong; the question is, when do you want to find out about disease? Would you prefer to find out ASAP when you can do something about it? Or at the end when it's too late?"

The good news is that given the advances in modern medicine, there are now therapeutics (drugs, supplements, foods, and lifestyles) that can be used to prevent and, in some cases, reverse heart disease, metabolic disease, and even dementia. Please look early when you have the greatest chance of taking successful action.

I call going through my annual Fountain Life upload: **"Not dying from something stupid,"** and I feel a great sense of confidence and relief when I complete any annual upload.

By the way, also under the category of "Not dying from something stupid," I also include: *wearing your seat belt, not texting while driving, and wearing a helmet when you ski.*

Fountain Digital & Fountain Health Benefits

I'll begin by admitting that APEX and EDGE membership are designed for those individuals who are looking for the *most advanced* diagnostics and therapeutics and those who desire access to *the best* longevity concierge physicians. As such, the price tag is significant (over $19.5K per year, including the concierge services and all testing).

Fountain Life uses the latest tech to diagnose illness early

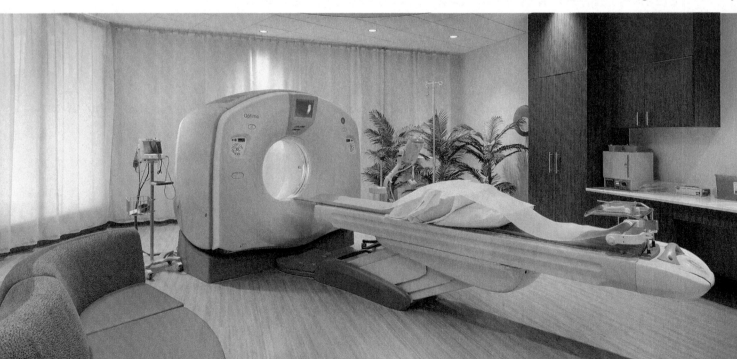

BUT, there are other options for those looking for something more affordable. Fountain has created 2 alternatives worth considering.

First, in 2024, Fountain Life is launching its much more affordable **Fountain Digital Membership**, enabling regular testing, telemedicine follow-up from one of Fountain's Functional Medicine MDs, wearables integration, along with a member dashboard and app.

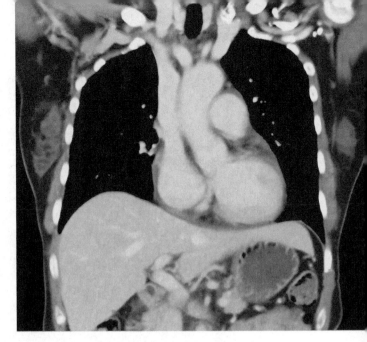
Fountain Life includes advanced imaging tech

Second, in 2022, Fountain launched **Fountain Health**, which is a health benefits offering for self-insurance companies with more than 50 employees. Fountain Health democratizes and demonetizes access to Fountain Services. The offering can mirror your company's current insurance plan in order to reduce employee disruption (same coverage, same copays, same deductibles). The primary benefit is that Fountain Health offers its members (your employees) *preventative testing* and coaching to find and prevent disease, saving lives and costs.

For more information on these programs, please check out **FountainLife.com** and **FountainHealth.com**.

What's Included in the Fountain Life APEX Upload?

The following is a more complete list of all the testing done at Fountain during an APEX and/or EDGE upload. All data is organized and evaluated by the company's AI systems and your Functional Medicine-trained longevity physician.

Imaging

- **Full Body & Brain MRI with AI Overlay:** This MRI imaging is used to generate a quantitative 3D visualization of your body, looking for tumors, masses, aneurysms, and other anomalies in the brain, neck, chest, kidneys, liver, spleen, pancreas, and other abdominal organs as well as the bladder, uterus, prostate, and other pelvic organs. The imaging also measures all brain structures, looking for white-matter lesions and any shrinkage. MRIs do not utilize radiation.

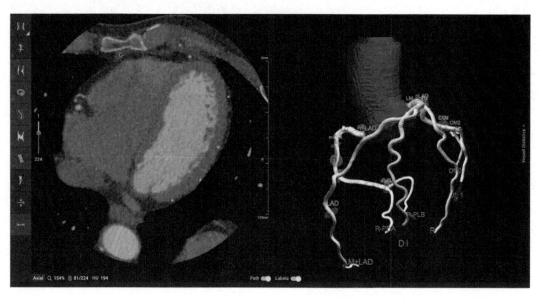

Cleerly uses AI to detect heart disease early

- **CCTA with AI Overlay**: This coronary computed tomography angiography , or CCTA, is used in intermediate-risk patients to evaluate for coronary artery disease. CCTAs use radiation and typically deliver a radiation dose in the range of 2 – 10 millisieverts (mSv). For comparison, on average, people are exposed to a background radiation dose of about 2 – 3 mSv per year from natural sources (such as cosmic radiation and radon), and a single chest X-ray typically exposes a person to about 0.1 mSv of radiation. Fountain Life uses a special type of AI overlay on their CCTAs called **Cleerly** that uniquely looks for soft plaque rather than calcified plaque. As it turns out, calcified plaque, which correlates with a calcium score, is stable and not concerning unless it forms a blockage. What can avulse and cause a heart attack is known as soft plaque, which is what the Cleerly scan is able to detect.

- **DEXA Whole Body Scan**: The DEXA, or "dual X-ray absorptiometry," scan is used to measure bone density (osteoporosis) and body composition (muscle and visceral fat). The DEXA is mainly used to detect osteoporosis or thinning of your bones and is recommended for women (primarily) and men who are 50 years old or older (especially if you have certain risk factors, such as having a parent who has broken a hip). The amount of radiation used in DEXA scans is very low and similar to the amount used in common X-rays.

- **Skin Cancer Screening:** This additional test is provided to help catch skin cancer early. For example, according to the American Cancer Society's estimates, approximately 97,610 new melanomas will be diagnosed in the United States in 2023 (about 58,120 in men and 39,490 in women). About 7,990 people are expected to die of melanoma (approximately 5,420 men and 2,570 women).

- **Retinal Scan:** With retinal imaging, Fountain Life can see symptoms of eye conditions that could not be detected before. Eye conditions such as diabetic retinopathy, glaucoma, age macular degeneration, and detached retina can be detected with retinal imaging. All these eye illnesses need quick medical care to prevent vision loss.

Genomics

- **Whole Genome Sequencing**: Decodes 100% of your DNA, all 6 billion letters, generating over 100GB of DNA data. In comparison, other genetic texts typically look only at certain areas of your genome and might only read as little as 0.02%.

- **Polygenic Risk Scores**: Once your full genome is sequenced, this test provides a measure of your risk for developing common chronic diseases, based on the total number of genetic changes related to the disease.

- **Single Nucleotide Polymorphisms Test (SNP)**: Identifies over 700,000 common genetic variations in your blood that affect everything from drug and toxin metabolism to efficiency of biochemical pathways.

- **Epigenetic "Age-Clock" Testing**: This epigenetic test looks at methylation markers on your DNA to predict your biological age in comparison to your chronological age and further determine how these changes will affect your body and overall health. It also determines your pace of aging (i.e., how fast you are aging each year).

Fountain Life's upload includes full-body scans

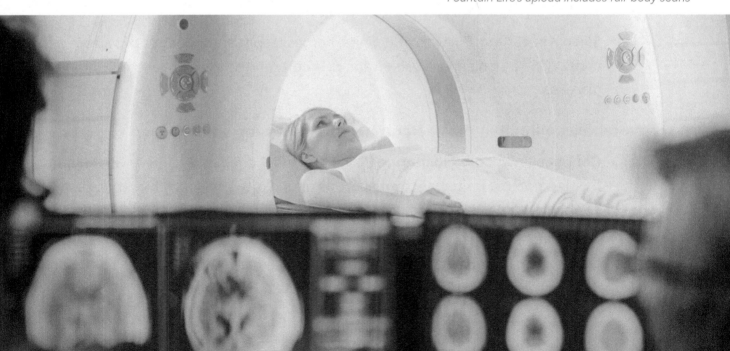

Blood Biomarkers, Cell-Free DNA & Toxins

- **100 Blood Biomarker Tests**: These tests contain an extensive and comprehensive set of clinical biomarkers looking at kidney and liver function; vitamin, mineral, and hormone levels; vascular and full body inflammatory markers; complete lipid and cholesterol panel; blood cell characterization; extensive metabolic health markers; autoimmune disease screening markers; cell membrane analysis; and a full set of heart disease risk factors.

- **Multi- Cancer Early Detection Blood Test:** This effectively finds cancers at early stages so they can easily be treated.

- **Toxins Testing**: Tests for the presence of environmental toxins which can cause acute or chronic toxic overload and may manifest in a variety of biological organ, tissue, and cellular-level dysfunctions.

This represents just a fraction of the testing I do every year at Fountain Life. Here's a partial list of the additional testing I do to understand what's going on inside my body:

- **Microbiome Sequencing**: Full Sequencing of your gut and oral microbiome.

- **Oral Pathogen Test**: Quantitative test for the most critical bacterial pathogens that confer the highest risk for infection, inflammation, cardiovascular, immune, and cognitive diseases.

- **Functional Movement Testing**: Using 2D motion capture and machine learning to assess human movement with pinpoint accuracy.

- **Strength Test**: Combination of upper and lower body strength measurements. Strength is a key indicator of overall longevity.

- **Sleep Apnea Test**: FDA-cleared digital home sleep test for obstructive sleep apnea (OSA). Undiagnosed sleep apnea is common and is a driver of all chronic diseases.

Metabolic, Mitochondrial & Neurocognitive Testing

- **Continuous Glucose Monitoring (CGM)**: As mentioned earlier, I love wearing my CGM to give me insight as to what foods or drinks will spike my blood glucose levels, giving me real-time glucose readings day and night.

- **Nutritional Test**: A blood and urine profile that evaluates over 125 biomarkers and assesses 40 antioxidants, vitamins, minerals, essential fatty acids, amino acids, and digestive support. It assesses all of the key metabolites in mitochondrial function.

- **Mitochondrial Function Test**: Testing lactic acid generated by a brief workout (treadmill or stationary bike) to determine your Zone 2 heart rate, estimate your VO2, and the presence of any mitochondrial dysfunction.

- **Neurocognitive Test**: A series of computerized neuropsychological tests to evaluate neurocognitive status and covers a range of mental processes from simple motor performance, attention, and memory, to executive functions. It also screens for mental health and mood disorders.

MyLifeforce

For those who are younger, and are focused on peak vitality, and perhaps don't have as much disposable income to spend on a full Fountain Life upload, there is another alternative called Lifeforce (mylifeforce.com).

In February 2022, when Tony Robbins and I wrote our book *Life Force: How New Breakthroughs in Precision Medicine Can Transform the Quality of Your Life & Those You Love*, we also started a company of a similar name called "Lifeforce" to provide a turnkey combination of comprehensive blood work, advanced nutraceuticals, hormone optimization protocols, and functional medicine support aimed at delivering a personalized blueprint for increasing vitality from the convenience of your home.

Lifeforce looks at 40+ biomarkers

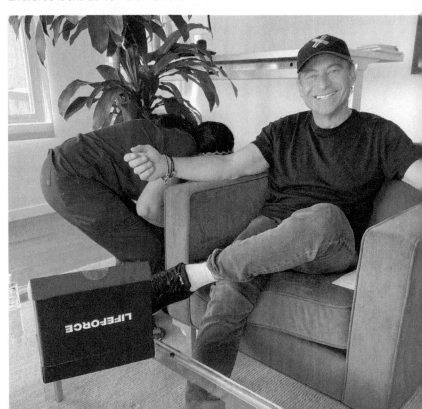

To personalize health, Lifeforce members get comprehensive blood work done every three months (with a phlebotomist sent to their home) looking at 40+ biomarkers to understand what's specifically driving someone's health status and performance, as evaluated by their personal dashboard and functional medicine support.

In just the first year, I'm happy to report that Lifeforce has improved the quality of life for *over 10,000 people*. Let's look at the data and key findings from our first 10,000 members:

- For male members aged 50 – 59, **51% have reported significant improvements in energy levels, libido, and sleep quality**.

- For female Lifeforce members aged 40 – 49, **55% reported better sleep quality and physical performance**.

In analyzing the data from Lifeforce members' first blood draws, there were 3 biomarkers that were most commonly out of optimal range:

- **Vitamin D**, which plays a crucial role in bone health, immune function, and overall health;

- **Testosterone**, which is important for both men *and* women because it helps energy levels, mood, and sexual function; and

- **DHEA (Dehydroepiandrosterone)**, a hormone that is a precursor to other hormones such as testosterone and estrogen.

- **One of the most consistent findings across all age groups was the improvement in testosterone**, specifically people getting into the optimal (not average or typical) range for their age group. For example, one statistic that stands out is that 48% of women between 60 – 69 years old got their testosterone into the optimal range in just three months using Lifeforce. (That certainly turns on its head that idea that your hormones only get worse as you age!)

Why This Matters

In 2004, my dear friend Ray Kurzweil wrote a milestone book called *Fantastic Voyage: Live Long Enough to Live Forever.*

In the book, Kurzweil describes three different "bridges" to get from now through to longevity escape velocity. *Bridge one* is a set of near-term life-extending solutions (e.g., a sugar-free diet and muscle-mass-increasing exercise) that should be followed until eventually *bridge-two interventions*—like cellular reprogramming, synthetic organs, and stem cell therapies—are safely and routinely available in the clinical setting. The third bridge, expected in the late 2030's involves the impact of nanotechnology when nanobots are available to repair your biology on an atomic basis.

Your job is to stay healthy and free of accidents long enough to intercept many of the bridge-two therapies expected later this decade.

Helping you cross *"bridge one"* is the goal of Fountain Life and Lifeforce and the content of this chapter.

If this is of interest to you, and I hope it is, check it out at **FountainLife.com** and **MyLifeForce.com**.

Fountain Life is a "Long-Life, Life-Long" Membership.

Fountain Life's Massive Transformative Purpose (MTP):

"Our MTP is to extend Member healthspan using the most advanced diagnostics and vetted personalized therapeutics."

Chapter Five:
Peter's Meds, Supplements, & Therapeutics

"It's likely that we're just another ten to twelve years away from the point that the general public will hit longevity escape velocity."

—Ray Kurzweil

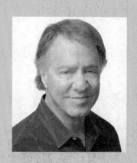

Peter's Legal Disclosure: *As I mentioned earlier in this book, I am an educator, entrepreneur, and scientist. I'm not a clinician and cannot make clinical recommendations for the prevention or treatment of any disease. In providing the details below, I am sharing the list of supplements and medications I'm taking based on my physician's recommendation.* **No one should start taking any supplement without first checking with his or her personal physician**. *Some supplements can be dangerous for people with certain pre-existing medical conditions and supplements can interfere with some prescription drugs. Supplements can also affect different people differently. The FDA has reviewed these supplements to determine whether their listed ingredients are safe to consume but no US regulatory authority has reviewed their ability to address cognition, dementia, Alzheimer's disease, or human brain health generally. The evidence of benefit for most of these supplements comes from laboratory experiments and/or from epidemiology data, not from human clinical trials. Supplements should only be purchased from trusted retailers and brands; testing has shown that many supplements are tainted with unlisted ingredients and/or do not contain the amount of the supplement listed on their label.*

My Prescription Medications

Note: The prescription medications listed below are specific to my medical objectives, based upon my blood biomarker testing (which I do on roughly a quarterly basis) and the recommendations of my Fountain Life physician. You will need to determine what is appropriate for you in consultation with your physician. My goal here is only to provide you with a full disclosure of my current regimen for informational purposes.

My Cholesterol Medications

One of my risks from family history and genetics is heart disease secondary to hypercholesteremia. As a result, the following is the cocktail of medications I take to give an ideal cholesterol blood panel. These work for me and keep my ApoB levels at an optimal range.

Zetia (10 mg): This is a combination medication used to treat high levels of cholesterol. Unlike other cholesterol-lowering agents, Ezetimibe works by selectively inhibiting the intestinal absorption of cholesterol and related phytosterols. This medication is taken orally daily.

Crestor (5 mg): I take Crestor (Rosuvastatin), a low-dose statin, for a number of reasons beyond its impact on lowering LDL (bad cholesterol) and triglycerides. It also has anti-inflammatory effects (established in various acute and chronic inflammatory models) as well as antiviral and antioxidant properties. It also helps to stabilize any vulnerable plaque. Other benefits of Crestor are that it is hydrophilic and doesn't cross the blood-brain barrier and, therefore, may not have an effect on neurocognition.

Repatha (PCSK9 biologic): This is a biologic medication (a monoclonal antibody) that is used to lower LDL cholesterol levels. It works by blocking a protein called PCSK9, which inhibits the liver's ability to remove LDL cholesterol from the blood. This is injected (with an autoinjector) every 2 weeks.

My "Longevity-related" Medications

1. Rapamycin (6mg) – taken once per week, on Sunday evening: Among the "longevity biohackers," the number one off-label therapeutic my colleagues are using is Rapamycin. Rapamycin is a compound discovered on Easter Island; it was initially used as an immune suppressant. It acts by inhibiting mTOR, a protein involved in cell growth and proliferation. For longevity, its benefits may come from the modulation of cellular processes such as autophagy (cellular "clean-up" mechanism) and metabolism. It has been found to extend the lifespan of multiple organisms. It is FDA-approved as an immune suppressant for use in organ transplants when taken daily. Taken once a week, it seems to be an immune modulator and has beneficial effects though its use in humans for longevity is still experimental. [**Rapamycin Dosing**: 0.1 mg/kg once weekly to be cycled for 3 months on and 1 month off, TruAge testing before and 6 months after].

Note: Before considering Rapamycin, it's crucial to consult with a qualified healthcare provider who can assess your individual health, risk factors, and potential benefits. Longevity research is still in its early stages, and there are many unknowns and risks associated with using drugs like Rapamycin for this purpose. Here are the known down-side complications: Rapamycin suppresses the immune system, which can make individuals more susceptible to infections. It can affect glucose metabolism and insulin sensitivity, potentially leading to insulin resistance and an increased risk of type 2 diabetes. Rapamycin use can cause side effects such as diarrhea, nausea, and vomiting, which may reduce the quality of life for some individuals. Long-term use of immunosuppressive drugs like Rapamycin has been associated with an increased risk of certain types of cancer, particularly skin cancer and lymphoma. The therapeutic can be hard on the kidneys, potentially leading to impaired kidney function, which can be problematic, especially for older individuals who may already have reduced kidney function. Also, Rapamycin can interact with other medications and may have different effects on different individuals.

2. CJC/Ipamorelin – Peptide to boost IGF-1/Growth Hormone, taken in a specific on-and-off cycle: These peptides stimulate the release of growth hormone (GH) from the pituitary gland, which in turn promotes the production of insulin-like growth factor 1 (IGF-1) in the liver. GH and IGF-1 can contribute to tissue repair, muscle growth, bone density, and improved metabolism. However, their role in longevity is complex as both low and high levels of IGF-1 have been associated with lifespan in various studies. (**Note**: As of the writing of this book, the FDA is conducting an extensive evaluation on Peptides and may restrict the sale of this class of therapeutics.)

3. Testosterone Optimization – twice per week: Testosterone optimization, often used as part of hormone replacement therapy, may have several benefits related to longevity. Adequate testosterone levels are associated with increased muscle mass, bone density, mood stability, cognitive function, and cardiovascular health. However, maintaining an optimal balance is crucial, as both low and high levels can have potential negative effects on health and longevity. Based on my lab levels, I take a 0.15ml injection twice per week.

My Nootropic Medication

I often fly around the world, and as much as I love getting 8 hours of sleep, many times when I'm crossing the continent or the globe and then need to go on stage, I will sometimes use a nootropic to focus my mind.

Nootropics, often referred to as "smart drugs" or "cognitive enhancers," are substances that aim to improve cognitive function, particularly executive functions like memory, creativity, or motivation, in healthy individuals.

While caffeine is a commonly used nootropic, I've reduced my intake to 1 cup (or less) of caffeinated coffee every 2 or 3 days. What I have found works very well for me is a prescription medication known as Modafinil (or Provigil) (my typical dose is 100 mg).

Modafinil is a medication that promotes wakefulness. It's most commonly used to treat sleep disorders such as narcolepsy, obstructive sleep apnea, and shift work sleep disorder. Despite its primary use, Modafinil has also gained popularity as a nootropic due to its potential to enhance cognition, particularly in terms of increasing alertness and reducing fatigue.

The exact mechanism of action of Modafinil is not fully understood. It's known to affect various neurotransmitters in the brain—chemicals that neurons use to communicate with each other. Some of the key neurotransmitters affected by Modafinil include dopamine, norepinephrine, histamine, and orexin (hypocretin).

Modafinil is thought to increase the availability of these neurotransmitters in parts of the brain that control wakefulness and alertness. For instance, it's known to inhibit the reuptake of dopamine, which increases the amount of dopamine available in the brain. This is a similar mechanism to some stimulants, but Modafinil doesn't tend to cause the same level of overstimulation or potential for addiction.

While Modafinil can be beneficial, and I've had no side effects myself, it's not without risks and potential side effects.

Note: *It's important to use Modafinil only under the guidance and supervision of a qualified healthcare provider, especially if you have underlying health conditions or are taking other medications. While it is generally considered safe and well-tolerated when used as prescribed, there are some potential downside risks associated with its use, including headache, nausea, nervousness, anxiety, gastrointestinal issues, and sleep disruption if taken too late in the day. Modafinil may cause increases in blood pressure and heart rate in some individuals. People with preexisting cardiovascular conditions should use it with caution and under medical supervision. While rare, Modafinil has been associated with psychiatric side effects such as mood changes, agitation, and, in rare cases, hallucinations. Modafinil should not be used when consuming alcohol. It's also important to remember that Modafinil doesn't replace the need for sleep.*

Modafinil is a medication primarily used to treat sleep disorders like narcolepsy, sleep apnea, and shift work sleep disorder.

My Skin Care

My favorite skin product is called OneSkin, a product I use every day, twice per day. OneSkin's product OS-1 addresses the root cause of skin aging, specifically senescent cells, which are damaged cells that build up in the body, contributing to aging and age-related diseases. As senescent cells accumulate in our skin, they create wrinkles and sagging, produce inflammation, and make us more susceptible to skin cancer. OS-1 is a 20 amino acid peptide. OneSkin's experiments have shown that this proprietary peptide can significantly decrease the level of senescent cells, reducing the age of the skin by several years at a molecular level.

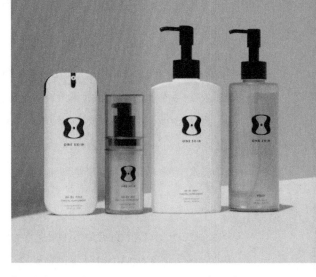

OneSkin's products can reverse skin's biological age

And yes, I also use an SPF 30 facial sun protection, especially on days when I'm out and about in the sun.

My Supplements

In addition to the Lifeforce supplements/products listed above, the following are supplements that I take as part of my longevity practices at various times depending on my medical test results. You can evaluate which are appropriate for you and at what dosages.

Creatine (morning of workouts): Creatine helps to generate ATP in skeletal muscles, which is the body's fuel source, it thus has been shown to enhance muscle strength, power, endurance, and exercise performance, which can contribute to maintaining overall physical function and mobility as we age, thereby promoting longevity. Since your body uses a lot of resources to make creatine, it can be helpful to take it to free up some of those resources.

Alpha Lipoic Acid: Alpha lipoic acid is a potent antioxidant that helps protect cells from oxidative stress. By neutralizing free radicals and supporting cellular, especially mitochondrial health, it may contribute to longevity by reducing the risk of age-related damage.

Selenomethionine: Selenomethionine is a form of selenium, a trace mineral that acts as an antioxidant and supports immune function. Adequate selenium levels have been associated with reduced risk of certain chronic diseases, potentially promoting longevity. You can usually get selenium from your food, but since many agriculture soils are deficient in selenium it can be important to supplement.

Lion's Mane: Lion's Mane is a mushroom with potential neuroprotective effects. It may support brain health by promoting the production of nerve growth factors and enhancing cognitive function, which could contribute to maintaining mental acuity and longevity.

Vitamin D with K2: Vitamin D plays a crucial role in bone health and immune function. When combined with vitamin K2, it helps ensure calcium is properly utilized and deposited in bones, potentially reducing the risk of fractures and supporting overall health as we age. Vitamin K2 has also been shown to reduce arterial stiffness by decreasing microcalcifications and lowering the incidence of diabetes and cardiovascular disease.

Seed/Probiotic (30 billion bacteria): A healthy gut microbiome is essential for various aspects of health. A high-quality seed/probiotic supplement with a diverse range of beneficial bacteria can help support digestion and immune function and potentially improve overall health and longevity.

CoQ10 with PQQ: Coenzyme Q10 (CoQ10) and Pyrroloquinoline quinone (PQQ) are both involved in cellular energy production and have antioxidant properties. These compounds may help protect mitochondria, the energy factories of cells, and support overall cellular health, potentially promoting longevity. Since statin drugs inhibit the enzyme that makes CoQ10 in our bodies, it is important to supplement with CoQ10 whenever taking a statin.

Quercetin: Quercetin is a flavonoid with antioxidant and anti-inflammatory properties. It may help reduce oxidative stress and inflammation and support cardiovascular health, which can contribute to overall longevity.

Xymogen (Methyl Protect): Xymogen's Methyl Protect is a supplement containing B vitamins designed to support methylation, a key biochemical process involved in gene expression and cellular function. By optimizing methylation, it may help promote overall health and potentially contribute to longevity.

Magnesium Threonate & Magnesium Glycinate: Magnesium is an essential mineral involved in numerous physiological processes. Magnesium threonate can get into the brain and thus has been suggested to enhance brain function and support cognitive health, while magnesium glycinate may help with relaxation and sleep. By promoting brain and overall well-being, they may indirectly contribute to longevity.

ProdromeNeuro & ProdromeGlia: ProdromeNeuro and ProdromeGlia are supplements designed to support brain health and protect against neurodegenerative conditions. By providing nutrients and compounds that promote brain function and reduce oxidative stress, they may help maintain cognitive vitality and potentially contribute to longevity.

Arterosil: Arterosil is a supplement that has been shown to regenerate the endothelial glycocalyx which is the protective lining inside all of our blood vessels. It thus supports endothelial function, which is important for maintaining healthy blood vessels. By promoting proper blood flow and reducing the risk of cardiovascular disease, Arterosil may contribute to overall longevity by supporting heart health.

Taurine: Taurine is amazing for mitochondrial health, mitochondrial proteostasis, nfr2 upregulation and MTP pore control. I take 1,000 mg per day, 5 days per week.

It's important to note that while these supplements have shown potential benefits, individual results may vary, and it's always recommended to consult with a healthcare professional before starting any new supplement regimen.

NAD+ Boosters: NMN, NR, and Nuchido TIME+

One group of supplements, NAD (nicotinamide adenine dinucleotide) boosters, deserve their own category in this chapter of the book. Before I share with you what I'm taking and why, allow me to provide you with some important background on NAD and why it's important to boost this particular molecule in your body.

Let's Begin with Sirtuins

Sirtuins are a set of 7 regulatory genes that have two different and competing functions in your cells. First, they govern the epigenome, turning the right genes on at the right time and in the right cell, boosting mitochondrial activity, reducing inflammation, and protecting telomeres. And second, they have another critical function in directing DNA repair.

As we age, the need for DNA repair increases because of accumulated damage. Makes sense, right? At age 20, we've only had a little exposure to environmental toxins and radiation, but by age 60, we have had three times the exposure, and because DNA damage accumulates, the need for repair is constantly increasing. As such, our sirtuins become overtaxed, frantically responding to one fire alarm after the next. As they focus on DNA repair, they get distracted from their second critical job of regulating the epigenome, deciding which genes should be turned on and which should be off.

The double-hit result? As we age and accumulate more and more DNA damage, our ability to repair the damage at the same time becomes more and more challenging. From entire organ systems down to individual cells, our bodies become dysregulated. Epigenetic noise accumulates. Genes that have no business being on are steadily switched on and vice versa. It's epigenetic mayhem!

In a nutshell, that's the dynamic of aging on a molecular level: the tension between gene regulation and gene repair and how we pay the price when our sirtuins become overwhelmed.

This leads us to another important question, for which the answer can combat the disease of human aging: how can we revive and supercharge our sirtuins?

The Answer is NAD+

Thanks in large part to Dr. David Sinclair's work at Harvard Medical School, we now know that our sirtuins can't do much of *anything*—including fixing our DNA—without a heaping helping of NAD+, a molecule that is critical to power the entire sirtuins system. So it's sobering to learn that we lose about half of our NAD+ by our 50s... right around the time when we need it more than ever to function at peak efficiency. Not only do our sirtuins have more and more work to do as we age, but they don't have enough NAD+ fuel to do their job!

Does this sound like a grim story to you? In fact, it's just the opposite. First, as we shall see in the next section, there is something you can do to aid your sirtuins in boosting your NAD+ levels. Second, if you've stayed with me this far, you should be ecstatic about this recent shift in scientific thinking. Unlike mutations in our genome, epigenetic aging is predictable and reproducible—and, based on recent clinical trials, possibly *reversible.*

NMN And Muscular Mice

In his research at Harvard, Dr. Sinclair conducted a remarkable experiment. His team gave NMN (nicotinamide mononucleotide), the precursor molecule converted into NAD+ inside our cells, to twenty-month-old mice (equivalent to a human in their 60s). The result was transformative, reviving their mitochondria and increasing their blood flow and the size and strength of their muscles. Within 2 months, the revitalized animals were running 60% further than an untreated control group. They'd become as vigorous as mice half their age. By every measurement that mattered, they were young again! This is why Sinclair personally takes a gram of NMN every morning as a supplement.

How I Supplement My NAD+

When I think about boosting my NAD+ levels, there are 3 approaches I've adopted:

The first approach is by taking oral NMN. Currently, I prefer a brand called Elevant Optima (Elevant.co), which comes in pleasantly tasting 125 mg chewable tablets. I first learned about Elevant from Dr. Eric Verdin, CEO of the Buck Institute. I will typically take between 750 and 1,000 mg per day.

Note: One company, Metrobiotech, is currently conducting human clinical trials of a crystalized version of NMN they have named MIB-626. These trials are looking at the impact of MIB-626 in a wide variety of indications ranging from increased muscle endurance and neurogeneration to treating COVID-related kidney failure and even heart failure. If Metrobiotech is successful in having NMN characterized as an FDA-regulated drug, then it will stop being sold as a supplement. Perhaps most interestingly, in July 2021, it was leaked that the U.S. Special Operations Command (SOCOM) has "completed preclinical safety and dosing studies in anticipation of follow-on performance testing" using Metrobiotech's MIB-626 molecule. "If the preclinical studies and clinical trials bear out, the resulting benefits include improved human performance, such as increased endurance and faster recovery from injury," said Navy Commander. Timothy A. Hawkins, a spokesperson for SOCOM. If all goes well with clinical trials, it's hoped that MIB-626 will gain regulatory approval as a new drug available to all of us by the end of 2025.

The second approach is by taking oral NR (nicotinamide riboside). NR is a naturally occurring form of vitamin B3 that can be converted into NAD+ in the body. Both NR and NMN are intermediates in the NAD+ biosynthetic pathway. That means they're both steps in the process the body uses to produce NAD+. So, they're closely related in that they both serve the goal of increasing NAD+ levels, though they do so through slightly different pathways. The leading supply of NR comes in a product called Basis by Elysium Health.

The third approach I use is a product called Nuchido TIME+. It boosts NAD+ levels through a combination of ingredients that work in synergy. Nuchido TIME+ activates the NAD+ recycling pathway by activating NAMPT, restoring the cell's natural ability to produce and recycle NAD+. Nuchido TIME+ also inhibits CD38, ensuring NAD+ is available for beneficial pathways. I take 3 capsules in the a.m. and 3 in the evening.

My Therapeutics (I'm Considering)

The following are the therapeutic protocols I am either participating in or investigating under the Fountain Life EDGE membership. Note some of these are still in development.

Senolytics Protocol – Senolytics are a class of drugs that selectively target and eliminate senescent cells, which are cells that have stopped dividing and are thought to contribute to aging and age-related diseases. There has been growing interest in senolytics as potential therapies for improving healthspan and lifespan. While the field is still emerging, several senolytic agents have gained attention for their potential longevity benefits:

1. **Dasatinib & Quercetin**: This combination is perhaps the most studied senolytic regimen. Dasatinib, originally an anti-cancer drug, and quercetin, a natural flavonoid found in many fruits and vegetables, have been shown in preclinical studies to selectively eliminate senescent cells in various tissues.

2. **Fisetin**: A natural flavonoid found in fruits like strawberries, fisetin has demonstrated senolytic properties in both cell culture and animal models.

3. **Spermidine**: A natural polyamine, spermidine has been shown to extend lifespan in various model organisms, possibly through autophagy activation and potential senostatic effects.

It's important to note that while many of these compounds show promise in preclinical studies, their efficacy and safety in humans, especially for long-term use, remain to be fully established. Clinical trials are underway for several of these agents to assess their potential as senolytic therapies in humans.

Exosomes – Exosomes are small vesicles containing growth and signaling factors produced by stem cells, used to communicate and stimulate repair and growth. Treatment with exosomes is a versatile and precisely targeted therapy that can be used to address conditions such as chronic pain, osteoarthritis, and musculoskeletal injuries. Currently, exosomes are not approved by the FDA and their use is investigational. I have used exosomes both locally (i.e., injection at sites of inflammation) and in my shoulder post-surgical repair of my rotator cuff. I've also used it to stimulate follicular growth on my scalp. Exosomes have also been used for an overall regenerative therapeutic when given intravenously. Today, exosomes are likely to be provided through Fountain Life under an Institutional Review Board (IRB) approved clinical trial.

Therapeutic Plasma Exchange (TPE) – Therapeutic plasma exchange is a medical procedure that removes and replaces the plasma in your blood. Plasma is the liquid part of blood that contains proteins, antibodies, and other substances. TPE is used to treat a variety of diseases, including autoimmune diseases, neurological disorders, hematological disorders, and poisoning (where TPE can remove toxins that have been ingested or inhaled). TPE is not a cure for any disease, but it can be used to improve symptoms and prolong life. There is some evidence that TPE may have pro-longevity benefits. It's also suggested that with aging, our blood accumulates harmful substances, which could possibly be removed with plasma exchange, potentially slowing down the aging process. For example, one study found that TPE increased the lifespan of mice by 30%. However, more research is needed to confirm these findings in humans.

The typical TPE protocol proposed by Dr. Dobri Kiprov (who pioneered much of this work) for longevity benefits is as follows:

- Frequency: The protocol calls for TPE to be performed once a week for a total of 12 weeks.

- Volume: Each TPE session removes 1.5 liters of plasma.

- Replacement fluid: The replacement fluid is a mixture of 5% human albumin and saline.

- Indication: The protocol is indicated for people who are interested in improving their healthspan and longevity.

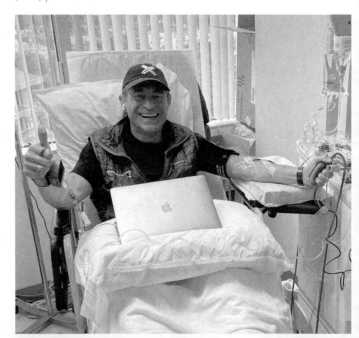

Peter receiving a Therpeutic Plasma Exchange (TPE) procedure

Dr. Kiprov believes that TPE can help slow the aging process by removing harmful proteins and other substances from the blood. He has conducted several studies that have shown that TPE can improve cognitive function, reduce inflammation, and increase lifespan in animals. Here are some of the potential benefits of TPE for longevity:

- Reduced inflammation: Inflammation is a major factor in aging and age-related diseases. TPE can help to reduce inflammation by removing harmful proteins and other substances from the blood.

- Improved cognitive function: TPE has been shown to improve cognitive function in animals and humans. This is likely due to the removal of harmful proteins that can damage brain cells.

- Increased lifespan: As mentioned above, several studies have shown that TPE can increase lifespan in animals. However, this has not yet been proven in humans.

Stem Cell Banking – Partnering with private, state-of-the-art facilities, Fountain Life is facilitating its members to participate in the collection, processing, and storing of their own fat-derived stem cells and bone marrow-derived stem cells.

Biobanking – Biobanking of serum, plasma, whole cells (WBC), microbiome, saliva, and urine. Partnering with a private, state-of-the-art biobank, Fountain Life will facilitate the process of collecting, processing, storing, and distributing various biological samples for future purposes.

The Power of Stem Cells

We are at the cusp of a stem cell revolution. Understanding and harnessing these unique cells may unlock breakthroughs in longevity and therapeutic solutions to all kinds of chronic diseases and regenerative opportunities.

Let's first begin by understanding the two major categories of stem cells. First are **autologous stem cells**, which are derived from you, typically from your fat or bone marrow, and then delivered back to you. In other words, this is about you receiving your own cells. Second are **allogeneic stem cells**, which are cells coming from someone else, a donor, many times from a newborn (either umbilical cord or placental stem cells).

It's important to know that today, the use of allogeneic stem cells (meaning stem cells from another individual, such as an umbilical cord-derived stem cell treatment) is not approved by the FDA and is therefore not legal in the United States. It is for this reason that many individuals travel to permissive jurisdictions such as Mexico, Antigua, Panama, or Costa Rica. After evaluating many venues for their level of medical and scientific safety, Fountain Life has directed many friends and family to the Regenerative Medicine Institute in Costa Rica (RMI-International.com), where they can gain access to allogeneic umbilical cord stem cells for joint repair and general IV infusion.

Note, in early 2024, Fountain Life expects to have approval through the FDA for an IND (investigational new drug) implementation of allogeneic placental stem cells (provided by Celularity) for the treatment of frailty (i.e., sarcopenia or muscle loss). Such treatments would take place at Fountain Life's Headquarters in Orlando, Florida, under the care of our medical staff and Celularity's research team.

What are Stem Cells?

Stem cells are undifferentiated cells that can transform into specialized cells such as heart, neurons, liver, lung, skin and so on, and can also divide to produce more stem cells. In a child or young adult, these stem cells are in large supply, acting as a built-in repair system. They are often summoned to the site of damage or inflammation to repair and restore normal function. But as we age, our supply of stem cells begins to diminish as much as 100 to10,000-fold in different tissues and organs.

In addition, stem cells undergo genetic mutations, which reduce their quality and effectiveness at renovating and repairing your body.

A useful analogy is to imagine your stem cells as a team of service technicians in your newly constructed mansion. When the mansion is new, and the technicians are young, they can fix everything perfectly. But as they age and reduce in number, your mansion goes into disrepair and eventually crumbles.

But what if you could restore and rejuvenate your stem cell population?

One option is to extract and concentrate your own autologous adult stem cells from places like your adipose (or fat) tissue. However, these stem cells are fewer in number and have undergone mutations from their original "software code."

Many scientists and physicians now prefer an alternative source, obtaining stem cells from the placenta or umbilical cord, the leftovers of birth. These stem cells, available in large supply and expressing the undamaged software of a newborn, can be injected into joints or administered intravenously to rejuvenate and revitalize.

One can think of these stem cells as chemical factories generating vital growth factors that can help to reduce inflammation, fight autoimmune diseases, increase muscle mass, repair joints, and even revitalize skin and grow hair.

Over the last decade, the number of publications per year on stem cell-related research has increased 40x. The global stem cell therapy market size was estimated at $11.22 billion in 2022, and it is projected to reach around $31.41 billion by 2030 and grow at a compound annual growth rate (CAGR) of 13.73% during the forecast period 2023 to 2030.

What Am I Doing About Stem Cells?

My focus is on two areas. First, I bank my own stem cells (even though they are 62 years old, they will never be younger than they are today!). I will bank both my fat stem cells as well as my mesenchymal (bone marrow-derived) stem cells. How or when will I use them? I'm not sure yet, but this is a service that will be available at Fountain Life. Also, there is ongoing research that indicates that "co-incubating" my 62-year-old stem cells with newborn stem cells can make my cells more youthful. (Note: I am so tempted to use the term euthanize, but I don't think that works in this case.)

The second thing I will do, once the FDA-IND is in place at Fountain Life Orlando, is pursue therapeutic treatment with Celularity's placental stem cells when possible.

Peptide Protocols (more details):

Under guidance from the Fountain Life Medical team, I sometimes use peptides. Peptides are short chains of amino acids, the building blocks of proteins. In medicine, peptides can be used as therapies for a variety of conditions. They are typically injected into the body, although other administration methods are also used. Peptides can serve a range of functions. Some act like hormones, and others like neurotransmitters. Many control and influence how our bodies react to diet and physical exercise. Following are the peptides I've used and/or am considering:

Note: In the U.S., at the time of this printing, the FDA is in the process of coming out with guidance regarding the safety and regulation of Peptides. Check with your longevity physicians on what is available and considered safe.

Peptide: BPC-157

BPC 157, composed of 15 amino acids, is a partial sequence of body protection compound (BPC) that is discovered in and isolated from human gastric juice. Experimentally, it has been demonstrated to accelerate the **healing of many different wounds, including tendons, muscles, nervous system, and superior healing of damaged ligaments**. Those who suffer from discomfort due to muscle sprains, tears, and damage may benefit from treatment with this peptide. It can also help aid skin burns to heal at a faster rate and increase blood flow to damaged tissues. Animal studies suggest that BPC-157 has strong anti-inflammatory activity.

Common Formulas & Protocols

- BPC-157 (10mg) Lyophilized Vial - 300mcg SQ injection nightly for 30 days.
- BPC-157 (500mcg) Capsule - One capsule daily for 30 days.
- BPC-157 (500mcg) Sublingual Troche - One troche daily for 30 days.

Peptide: Selank

Selank is a synthetic peptide that was developed by the Institute of Molecular Genetics of the Russian Academy of Sciences. It's based on a naturally occurring immunomodulatory peptide called tuftsin, which plays an important role in immune system responses. Selank is known for its potential nootropic and anxiolytic (anti-anxiety) effects. It has been studied for its potential to improve anxiety, enhance cognitive functions, and modulate the immune system. Here are some specific areas of research:

1. **Anxiety and depression**: Selank has been studied for its potential to reduce anxiety and symptoms of depression. It appears to modulate the expression of GABA, which is one of the main inhibitory neurotransmitters in the human brain.

2. **Cognitive function**: Some research has suggested that Selank could improve cognitive function. It's thought that it may enhance memory and learning ability, though more research is needed in this area.

3. Immune modulation: Selank is derived from the peptide Tuftsin, which is known to modulate the immune system. As such, Selank may also have immune-modulating properties.

Common Formulas & Protocols

- Selank (7500mcg/ml) Nasal Spray 3ml Bottle - 750mcg (1 spray) each nostril daily.

Peptide: Semax

Semax increases brain-derived neurotrophic factor (BDNF) levels. BDNF is among the most active neurotrophins, which are chemicals that help to stimulate and control neurogenesis, the birth of new neurons in the brain. BDNF has been shown to play a role in neuroplasticity, which allows nerve cells in the brain to compensate for injury and adapt to new situations or changes in the environment. Basically, BDNF helps to support the survival of existing neurons and encourages the growth, regeneration, and creation of new neurons and synapses.

The understood benefits of Semax include: Improvement of cognitive function, improving long and short-term memory, helping to manage depression, improving non-proliferative diabetic neuropathy recovery from stroke/hypoxia, and improving glaucoma optic neuropathy. Semax may also be helpful in the treatment of PTSD and ADHD neuroprotection.

Common Formulas & Protocols

- Semax (7500mcg/ml) Nasal Spray 3ml Bottle - 750mcg (1 spray) each nostril daily.

Peptide: CJC-1295 / Ipamorelin

CJC 1295 is often prescribed by physicians as a growth hormone-releasing hormone (GHRH) analog. CJC 1295 has been shown to increase growth hormone as well as IGF-I secretion, and it has been able to do so in very large amounts. CJC 1295 stimulates growth hormone secretion and will keep a steady increase of HGH and IGF-1 with no increase in prolactin, leading to fat loss and increased protein synthesis, thereby promoting growth. We suggest using the CJC 1295 in combination with Ipamorelin as it provides a synergistic effect, generating five times the benefits of using the CJC 1295 or Ipamorelin alone. The combination allows for maximized release of GH because the CJC 1295 and Ipamorelin have different mechanisms of action and work on different receptors (GHRH-R & Ghrelin-R).

Subcutaneous administration of CJC 1295 resulted in sustained, dose-dependent increases in GH and IGF-I levels in healthy adults and was safe and relatively well tolerated, particularly at doses of 30 or 60 ug/kg. There was evidence of a cumulative effect after multiple doses.

"It is health that is the real wealth, and not pieces of gold and silver."

—Mahatma Gandhi

Chapter Six:
Peter's Longevity Mindset

"The best way to enjoy your aging process is to take care of your body and mind, to keep learning and growing, and to find joy and purpose in the present moment."

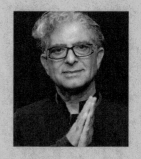

—Deepak Chopra, MD

What is a Longevity Mindset?

One of the most important elements of my Longevity Practices is creating and maintaining a Longevity Mindset.

A Longevity Mindset is one in which you believe in the ability of science to extend your healthspan, perhaps by 10 or 20 years. Further, it is a belief (and an understanding) that during these additional decades, science isn't standing still. Instead, health technologies are accelerating exponentially, continuing to make breakthroughs driven by AI, genome sequencing/editing, epigenetic modification, and gene therapy—all of which are being focused on expanding healthspan and reversing disease.

A Longevity Mindset means becoming the "CEO of your own health" and recognizing that "Life is short until you extend it."

What Shapes Your Longevity Mindset and Your Healthspan?

How long you live is a function of many factors: where you were born, your genetics, your diet, *and* your mindset. Most people imagine that longevity is mostly inherited, that the genetic cards you are dealt have predetermined your lifespan.

As I mentioned in the introduction and am repeating here to make a crucial point, **you may be surprised by the truth.**

In 2018, after the analysis of a 54-million-person ancestry database, scientists announced that lifespan has little to do with genes.

Your DNA is not your destiny

In fact, **heritability is accountable for only ~7% of your longevity**.

Other studies peg this somewhat higher, estimating that heritability accounts for some 20% or 30% of your lifespan—which still means, at a minimum, that lifestyle choices account for 70% of your longevity.

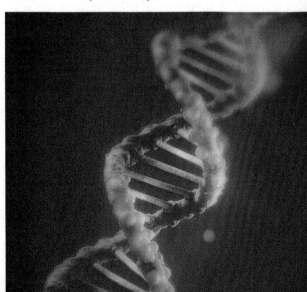

The power of shaping your healthspan is much more in your hands than you might have imagined. While we've already discussed things like diet, exercise, and sleep, one of the biggest (underestimated) impacts on your healthspan is your mindset, which we'll explore below.

There are 7 key mindset and lifestyle areas (under your control) that fundamentally impact your healthspan. Let's review each area together, and as we do, I invite you to ask yourself: *Where do I truly stand in this area? Where can I improve? What would it take for me to modify my beliefs and actions?*

#1. What do you honestly believe about your healthspan? Understanding your ingrained beliefs about your expected healthspan is the first place to begin. At one end of the spectrum, you see life as short and precious—you'll consider yourself lucky if you make it to 75 or 80 years old. At the other end, you're focused on breaking through 100 years old with energy and passion, making "100 years old the new 60."

In this latter mindset, you see aging as a disease that can be slowed, stopped, and perhaps even reversed.

#2. What media are you consuming? The type of content you consume (e.g., books, blogs, movies, news) constantly shapes how you think and directly impacts your Longevity Mindset. Are you reading the obituaries of old friends? Or are you reading books like *Life Force*, David Sinclair's *Lifespan*, or Sergey Young's *Growing Young*? Are you reading digital content about the latest political battle, or are you reading LongevityInsider.org, a free, **AI-enabled longevity newsletter** that summarizes daily breakthroughs and innovations from around the world?

Your mindset and lifestyle greatly affect your longevity

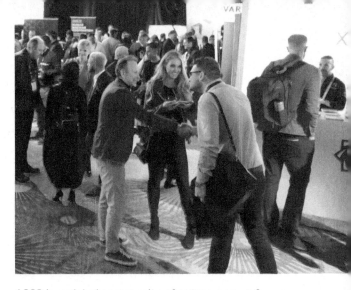

A360 is a global community of entrepreneurs & leaders changing the world

#3. Who do you hang out with? Who makes up your community? The people you spend time with have perhaps the biggest impact on shaping what you believe and the actions you take. Are you actively building and deeply engaging with a community that is optimistic and youthful despite their age? A group actively pursuing longevity, sharing best practices, and encouraging one another? A group that exercises together on a regular basis?

#4. Are you prioritizing sleep? Sleep is a fundamental tool to optimize your healthspan. As I've mentioned, a great book that details this is *Why We Sleep* by Dr. Matt Walker. We physiologically *need* 8 hours of sleep per night. Do you believe the motto that "There's plenty of time to sleep when I'm dead"? Or do you prioritize sleep and use the best available techniques to help you achieve 8 healthy hours of sleep?

#5. How healthy is your diet? There is truth to the saying, "You are what you eat." Do you eat whatever you want, whenever you want? Are you overweight and eating way too much sugar? Or have you intentionally shaped your diet, minimizing sugars and high glycemic foods while eating a diet high in whole plants and sufficient protein to build muscle?

#6. How much exercise do you get? Along with your mindset, sufficient sleep, and a healthy diet, exercise is fundamental to longevity. The latest research on longevity makes it clear that maintaining and (if possible) increasing muscle mass is critical. So, where are you on the exercise spectrum? On the one end, you don't exercise at all. On the other end, you're getting in 10,000 steps a day and are exercising with weights at least 3 times each week, focusing on interval training and weightlifting.

#7. Annual diagnostic upload? Most of us are optimists about our bodies. But in reality, we have no idea what's really going on internally—until that moment when we end up in the hospital with some condition. Your job is to catch any illness (cancer, inflammatory disease, insulin resistance, etc.) as early as possible when it is most easily reversed. The best way to do this is to make use of the increasingly available onslaught of diagnostic technologies that can help you find disease at inception.

Over the years, I've held a high-end, 5-day Abundance Platinum Longevity Trip where I bring together investors and family offices on a deep-dive into the entrepreneurs, scientists, and CEOs transforming this industry. Over the course of the 5 days, participants hear from over 50 leaders in the field in areas ranging from sleep and diet to stem cells and gene therapies.

At the beginning of the Trip, and then again at the end, I have them take a self-assessment on their Longevity Mindset. Here it is for you. For each of the 5 Mindset Areas, rate yourself 1 through 10 and then add up your score; the maximum is 50.

Your mindset is your most important asset. How do you score?

Mindset Areas	1 — 2 — 3	4 — 5 — 6	7 — 8 — 9 — 10	Day 1 Score	Day 5 Score
Overall Longevity Mindset (What I believe)	Life is short & precious. I hope to make it to 75.	I'm aiming to get to at least 80 yrs old, maybe to 100. My goal is to stay out of a wheelchair!	I will get past 120 yrs old (min) (healthy & fit). Shooting for a 150-year lifespan or older!		
What I Read & Watch (What I let into my brain)	I don't monitor what I read or watch. Typically I'm watching CNN /Fox, sometimes reading the obituaries of old friends.	I watch some negative news. I try to read more inspiring blogs & books and educate myself about the latest health and biotech breakthroughs.	I actively shape my Longevity Mindset by consuming inspiring Books (e.g., *Lifespan*) & Blogs & News (*Longevity Insider*).		
My Community (Who I hang out with)	I mostly hang out with older people who are always talking about disease, aches, pains and death.	I maximize my time with friends and loved ones, both young and old. We discuss diet, exercise and health, but not longevity.	My friends and I are young, or young-minded; We pursue longevity content and hang out with health-conscious individuals.		
My Diet, Sleep & Exercise (How I treat my body)	I eat whatever I want; I don't prioritize sleep, and rarely exercise. My health is not a top priority.	I know sleep, diet and exercise are important. I'm working on prioritizing these areas and learning about best practices.	I sleep 7+ solid hours per night. I am focused on building muscle mass and a healthy diet with Intermittent Fasting and No Sugar.		
My knowledge of cutting edge Diagnostics & Biotech Interventions	I have no idea what's going on inside my body. For my health I occasionally imbibe red wine & scotch. I'm not concerned.	My health strategy involves: (i) an annual check up, (ii) statins, (iii) BP medicine & (iv) Cardiac Score. I do what my doctor orders.	I have sequenced my genome, do an annual MRI; I take peptides, stem cells, exosomes, and the latest regenerative treatments, and joined a longevity team (e.g., Fountain Life).		
			Total Scorecard		

Why Your Mindset Matters: The "Will to Live"

I want to close this Longevity Mindset chapter with a notion about the power of the human mind. Specifically, "the will to live."

It's all about "mind over physiology."

A key mindset for longevity involves being excited about the future and having something to live for and look forward to.

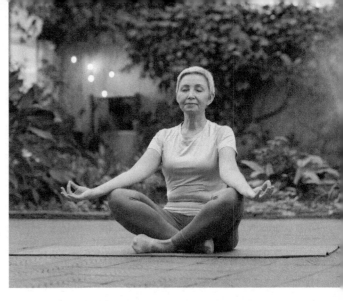

Meditation & mindfulness are key techniques for managing stress

My coach, Dan Sullivan of Strategic Coach®, puts it this way, "Always make your future bigger than your past."

Tony Robbins says, "Having a bigger purpose to live for is absolutely key to longevity."

My favorite story illustrating this comes from the annals of American history. As it turns out, in an extraordinary demonstration of "the will to live," two of America's Founding Fathers, Thomas Jefferson and John Adams, both willed themselves to live long enough to see the 50th anniversary of the Declaration of Independence.

Even though in the early 1800s the average life expectancy was only 44 years, Jefferson (who was 83) and Adams (who was 90) made it to July 4, 1826, *both dying on that exact date*, the 50th anniversary of the nation they had founded.

Clearly, they had a goal in mind, something to live for.

So, how long do you think you'll live? Until you're 80 years old? Maybe 100?

What mindset or purpose would you require to set a target of 120 healthy years and make it there?

Your health is your greatest wealth, and today is the most extraordinary time to be alive.

Please begin to change how you discuss your lifespan (and healthspan) with others. Make it known to friends and family (with conviction) that you're shooting for 100, 120, or even 156. Pick a number that inspires you and program that into your mind.

One of the most important conversations you can have with yourself, your friends, and loved ones is to ask the following question:

"What would you do with an extra 30 years of healthspan?"

Having a clear vision and emotionally connecting on why that is important to you makes all the difference in the world. *The results are powerful.*

For me, my motivations for getting an extra 30 years of healthspan are many, but primarily:

1. I had kids later in life (twin boys born when I was 50). I want to see them thrive and meet my grandkids and great-grandkids.

2. I want to see humanity settle the Moon (and go there myself), reach Mars, build O'Neil colonies, and settle space. I'm a child of the 60s when the Apollo program and that scientific documentary *Star Trek* showed us how far humanity can reach. I want to see it all.

3. I'm excited to see how the development of brain-computer interfaces proceeds, helps pioneer our ability to connect our consciousness with the cloud, and even pioneers the ability for humans to "upload" our minds. (Yes, I know this is pretty far out, but heck I'm 62, and a lot can happen in the next 60-plus years!)

Optimists Live Longer

I'll close with a compelling piece of data on why you should be optimistic about an extended healthspan, and why you should be optimistic in general.

In a study of 69,744 women and 1,429 men, published in the prestigious journal *Proceedings of the National Academy of Science*, it was found that **optimistic people live as much as 15% longer than pessimists.** The study was conducted over the course of 3 decades, controlling for health conditions, behaviors like diet and exercise, and other demographic information.

There is a lot to be grateful for and a lot under your control.

> "In a study of 69,744 women and 1,429 men, published in the prestigious journal Proceedings of the *National Academy of Science*, it was found that **optimistic people live as much as 15% longer than pessimists.**"

XPRIZE Healthspan: A Reason For Optimism

One of the most successful organizations I founded some 30 years ago is called the XPRIZE Foundation. XPRIZE is a nonprofit dedicated to inspiring and incentivizing breakthroughs in the most critical challenges facing humanity. The organization has been building a vision of hope and abundance for humankind's future by harnessing the power of innovators, technology, and resources to solve grand challenges.

 XPRIZE designs, funds, and launches large-scale incentive competitions to inspire breakthroughs in areas that are stuck or moving too slowly. Its competitions are funded by leading entrepreneurs, corporate giants and global philanthropists like Google (funder of the $30M Google Lunar XPRIZE), Elon Musk (funder of the $100M Carbon Removal XPRIZE and $15M Global Learning XPRIZE), Wendy Schmidt (funder of multiple oceans related XPRIZEs) and Ratan Tata (funder of the Water Abundance XPRIZE).

By conducting incentive prize competitions, XPRIZE enables human capital to create bold and transformative solutions that are scalable and drive real impact.

In the last 25 years, XPRIZE has launched 27 Competitions with $300M+ worth of cumulative prize purses. Of these 27 XPRIZEs, 19 have been awarded, 5 are still active, 1 competition was canceled, and 2 XPRIZEs were not won before their deadline.

By early 2024, an additional $250M worth of XPRIZEs (currently in development) will be launched. Historically, the payoff to humanity from these competitions has been huge—typically 20x – 30x the purse is spent cumulatively by the teams in their effort to win the prize. Here's one example from our first-ever competition:

$10M Ansari Spaceflight XPRIZE: The Ansari $10M XPRIZE was designed to lower the risk and cost of going to space by incentivizing the creation of a reliable, reusable, privately financed, crewed spaceship that finally made private space travel commercially viable. Teams around the world were challenged to build a reliable, reusable, privately financed, manned spaceship capable of carrying 3 people to 100 km, above the Earth's surface twice within 2 weeks.

On October 4, 2004, Mojave Aerospace Ventures won the $10M Grand Prize for their SpaceShipOne. Led by famed aerospace designer Burt Rutan and his company Scaled Composites, with financial backing from Paul Allen, the team's winning technology was licensed by Richard Branson to create Virgin Galactic. With the awarding of this competition, a brand-new multi-billion private space industry was launched.

XPRIZEs work, they recruit hundreds of teams, each trying different approaches.

So why should we be optimistic about extending the human healthspan? And why is extending the human healthspan beneficial to society? Consider the following...

$101M XPRIZE Healthspan: On November 29, 2023, the XPRIZE Foundation is launching its largest-ever XPRIZE ($101 million), one focused on "Extending Healthspan" in humans. This competition will run between 2023 and 2031, and in success will help drive new breakthroughs in the field, attract significant capital, drive public attention, and help accelerate the regulatory frameworks required to slow, stop, or even reverse aging.

The Global Impact Of Increased Healthspan

"We show that a **slowdown in aging that increases life expectancy by 1 year is worth US$38 trillion, and by 10 years, US$367 trillion.** Ultimately, the more progress that is made in improving how we age, the greater the value of further improvements."

—*Nature Aging* (Jul 5, 2021)

Chapter Seven:
Women's Health

"*People are always asking me, 'What do you want people to say about you in a hundred years from now?' I always say I want them to say, 'Dang, don't she still look good for her age?'*"

—Dolly Parton

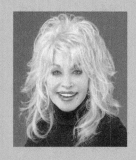

Dr. Helen's Longevity Practices

By Helen Messier, PhD, MD

Chief Medical & Scientific Officer, Fountain Life

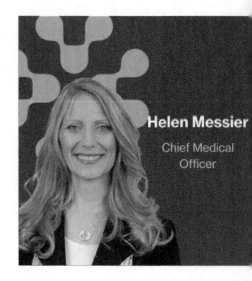

Helen Messier

Chief Medical Officer

Peter asked me to add a chapter on women's health in addition to his excellent advice and longevity practices outlined in the previous chapters.

Before sharing details on what I personally do to extend my healthspan, I think it's important to explain why women, in general, need their own set of longevity practices.

Simply put, women are different from men.

Physiologically, women, of course, are the ones who carry the babies, and we have all the physical characteristics that help us give birth and remain healthy. We have higher levels of body fat to provide the necessary stores of fat to manage pregnancy and breastfeeding. There are huge hormonal differences between men and women. From a cardiovascular perspective, our hearts and blood vessels are smaller in size, and we have smaller lung volumes. Even our bones tend to be less dense.

Based on these physiological differences, women have unique health concerns. Gynecological cancers, menopause, pregnancy—these are all, of course, unique to women. But there are also diseases that tend to affect women more than men: Alzheimer's disease, depression, autoimmune diseases, and stroke are all more common in women. One reason for the difference in disease prevalence is that women's and men's immune responses are quite different. Women tend to have a more robust immune response for both innate (early) and adaptive (late) immunity.[1] This results in women having lower rates of cancer (1 in 3 vs 1 in 2 for men), but also higher rates of inflammation and autoimmune disease.[2]

---

[1] *Sabra L Klein and Katie L Flanagan, "Sex Differences in Immune Responses," Nature reviews. Immunology, August 22, 2016, https://pubmed.ncbi.nlm.nih.gov/27546235/.*

[2] *Heather M. Derry et al., "Sex Differences in Depression: Does Inflammation Play a Role?," Current Psychiatry Reports 17, no. 10 (October 15, 2015), https://doi.org/10.1007/s11920-015-0618-5.*

Unfortunately, despite a universal understanding that there are anatomical and physiological differences between men and women, there is a significant gap in the number of studies that actively explore or at least take into account these differences. For example, in 1977, the FDA guidelines advised that women of childbearing potential should be excluded from all drug trials. Although women are now included in clinical trials of drugs, devices, and biologics, there is sparse understanding of whether outcomes are different between men and women. Of the drugs that have been taken off the market, 80% had greater adverse effects in women.

Even basic science research is lacking in women. For example, although hormones like estrogen have a profound effect on the brain, less than 0.5% of neuroimaging literature takes this into account, and only 10% of immune studies analyze data by sex despite the enormous effects sex plays in immune function.

So, for the women reading this, simply acknowledging and understanding that we are different from men—both physiologically and in terms of our unique health concerns—is critical to understanding how to extend our healthspans. It's also empowering, allowing us to act on what we do know while, at the same time, acknowledging that we still have much to learn.

That's the rationale and spirit behind sharing my own longevity practices: to provide a helpful guide for other women to extend their lifespans and health spans while considering their unique physiology and health concerns.

So, the following discussion of several longevity practices, specifically for women, covers a variety of topics from hormones and fasting to toxins and stress.

Hormones

The Importance of Taking a Holistic Approach to Hormone Balance & Replacement

Every woman is familiar with the negative effects of hormones—from mood swings and fatigue to weight gain. These effects occur when our hormones are not in balance.

Yet, hormones do not only cause problems for women, but they are also essential for optimal health. Not only do the hormones estrogen and progesterone make us female and facilitate pregnancy and childbirth, they are responsible for maintaining brain, bone, heart, blood vessel, urinary, skin, hair, and breast health, to name a few. In fact, there are estrogen receptors on almost every cell in our bodies. A recent study even showed that our brains remodel themselves in sync with our menstrual cycle, where high estrogen and low progesterone levels, as found in midcycle, drive the expansion of areas of the brain needed for episodic memory and spatial cognition. And when we lose our hormones during menopause, we feel the effects of hot flashes, night sweats, vaginal dryness, weight gain, hair and skin changes, and even brain fog. Once a woman hits menopause, she is also at increased risk for osteoporosis, cardiovascular disease, dementia, metabolic diseases, and cancers.

Recently, there has been a lot of discussion about hormone replacement for peri- and post-menopausal women and a variety of theories touting different approaches. What are optimal levels of estrogen? Which hormone replacement strategy is best?

But we need to remember that the process of optimally managing our hormones as women involves much more than measuring levels of hormones like estrogen and progesterone. It means understanding how our bodies naturally produce hormones, our monthly cycles, how our hormone receptors are expressed in our cells, and even how we metabolize hormones. In this section, I will summarize the key points about these important topics and briefly share the hormone replacement approach I use personally and with my patients.

What Optimal Hormone Balance Looks Like

As women, when we think about longevity and replacing hormones, we shouldn't fight nature. We need to consider what normally happens in our bodies, and even more importantly, we need to ensure we're not doing things differently than what our bodies are naturally optimized for.

So, what is optimal hormone balance?

The first thing to understand is our hormones cycle—they don't stay at the same levels throughout a given month. In fact, there is an intricate feedback loop controlled by the hypothalamus in our brain, which sends signals down to our pituitary gland and then to our ovaries to produce estrogen and progesterone. This leads to positive and negative feedback loops that control our hormone levels.

The results of this process are the monthly, cyclical changes in hormones that we experience as women. During the first few days of the month, both estrogen and progesterone are at low levels, and then our estrogen levels tend to rise midway through the month (the ovulatory phase) before dropping precipitously. And just as our estrogen drops, our progesterone levels go up. This cycling of hormones causes the build-up of the endometrial lining and subsequent shedding resulting in our monthly period.

So, our estrogen and progesterone levels vary at different times—this cycle is completely natural and normal.

Why is this important to understand for hormone replacement?

Because when your estrogen levels peak around midway through the month, this serves as a signal to your estrogen receptors, progesterone receptors, and even your testosterone receptors to be expressed. And that's critical because any hormone you take isn't going to work if it can't bind to a receptor. So, if you have low levels of estrogen, then your body won't have the signal to get each of your receptors ready to interact with whatever hormone you're taking.

Here's the key thing to remember: If we understand the natural cycle of our bodies and how they produce hormones and mimic as closely as possible what our bodies do naturally, then we will be much more effective at reaching optimal hormone balance. Because, for example, if you tend to give estrogen and progesterone together at the same time, in the same dose, every day, then over time, your receptors will down-regulate and the hormones won't have as much of an impact. This applies to receptors for all sex hormones, including estrogen, progesterone, and testosterone.

My Own Approach to Hormone Replacement

When I give hormones to women, I focus on physiological hormone replacement. This is designed to mimic as closely as possible a normal menstrual cycle with the continuously changing levels of hormones followed by a withdrawal bleed. Again, I want to mimic a natural cycle—not go against it. For that reason, I don't give continuous, combined hormones. Continuous combined HRT is the most popular, where estrogen and progesterone are given at the same dose every day. There is no cycling and no withdrawal bleed.

While simplicity and lack of bleeding make this a popular method, my experience has been that it tends to stop working overtime, and women no longer experience the beneficial effects. This is likely due to the downregulation of their hormone receptors. In many cases, I do not even need to give testosterone replacement since it results in an upregulation of testosterone receptors, and the small amount that is still made by our adrenal glands is enough for many women. In some cases, it will still be necessary.

Now, I will acknowledge that the physiological hormone replacement approach is a bit more involved (e.g., you must use two creams twice per day) and adjust the dosage according to the day of the month. In my experience, if you stick with this process for about 3 months, then you will start to notice a difference and positive changes. Hormone levels should be measured in the blood to ensure you take the right dosage; however, the energy and vitality that women feel is a sure sign you are on the right track.

Understanding How Hormones Are Metabolized

During our natural cycles, as well as when we take hormones, we metabolize them and get rid of the used hormones in our urine and in our stool. In fact, hormone production and metabolism is an intricate, beautifully orchestrated dance that responds to our needs. For example, if we are under a lot of stress, our body will direct hormone production towards making the cortisol we need rather than progesterone or estrogen. This is why some women stop cycling when they are under a significant amount of stress.

Let's take a closer look at the amazing dance of our sex hormones. Our bodies start with a "mother" hormone called pregnenolone, which is made from cholesterol. (In fact, one of the reasons we need cholesterol is that all of our hormones are made from it.) Pregnenolone then goes on to make DHEA, which then produces testosterone and other androgens. As I pointed out above, women also need testosterone, and we also have testosterone receptors. Estrogen is, in fact, from testosterone in both men and women.

Then, we have different types of estrogen (E1, E2, E3), and each of these has different effects—they bind the estrogen receptors with different levels of strength that results in different effects. Once they have completed their job, these estrogens are then metabolized in order for our body to dispose of them.

To explain further, it's important to understand that estrogen isn't just one hormone; it's a class of hormones. There are 3 major types of estrogen that are naturally found in the human body, and each serves slightly different roles:

1. Estrone (E1) is a weak estrogen, and in women who are no longer menstruating, it's the primary estrogen present. It's mainly produced in the fat tissues, especially after menopause. In pre-menopausal women, estrone plays a more minor role. However, after menopause, it becomes more significant as the primary type of estrogen in the body.

2. Estradiol (E2) is the most potent and predominant form of estrogen found in reproductive-age women and is produced in the ovaries. Estradiol is responsible for the development of female secondary sexual characteristics and the regulation of the menstrual cycle. It also plays a vital role in many other bodily functions, including maintaining bone density and affecting heart and brain health.

3. Estriol (E3) is a weak estrogen primarily associated with pregnancy, produced in large amounts by the placenta during pregnancy. Estriol helps to prepare the uterus for the developing fetus and supports the placenta and amniotic sac throughout gestation. In non-pregnant women, estriol levels are relatively low.

In general, the balance and levels of these hormones change over a person's lifetime, especially during significant life events like puberty, menstruation, pregnancy, and menopause. Monitoring and understanding these levels can be crucial in certain medical contexts.

Depending on our genetics and nutritional status, how we metabolize our hormones can be quite variable. Estrogen can preferentially be metabolized down one of the given pathways versus another, resulting in the production of either non-toxic hormone metabolites or more dangerous hormone metabolites that can cause DNA damage. For example, many women with breast cancer tend to make a lot of 4-Hydroxy estrogen metabolite, which damages DNA.

When we replace our hormones, it is important to monitor our levels and types of estrogen metabolites to make sure we get all the benefits of hormone replacement without causing any harm. The main enzymes involved in regulating estrogen metabolism are the P450 enzyme system (CYP19A1, CYP1A1, CYP1B1), the COMT enzyme, which uses methyl groups, as well as sulfation and glucuronidation. The interesting thing is that these enzymes are coded for by genes that have significant variability in different people. That is, we are all born with a different ability to metabolize our hormones. In addition, nutrients such as sulforaphane from broccoli and curcumin found in turmeric can regulate how well these enzymes work. Other nutrients such as DIM and I3C that come from cruciferous vegetables can actually lower the amount of estrogen in your body.

Another often overlooked but essential component of hormone balance is regulated by the gut microbiome. We have trillions of microorganisms, such as bacteria and viruses, that live in our gut, and they have an impact on almost all aspects of our health, including our hormones. Dysbiosis, which is an imbalance in our gut bacteria as well as a reduction of microbe diversity, has an impact on the estrobolome. The estrobolome is the collection of bacteria in the gut that can metabolize and thus modulate the amounts of circulating estrogen. Thus, our gut microbiome can have a profound impact on our hormone levels.

For example, things like decreased microbe diversity or inflammation can affect the levels of β-glucuronidase activity. β-glucuronidase is an enzyme made by our gut microbes that can eliminate the glucuronide tag our liver uses to dispose of estrogen and allow for the estrogen to get reabsorbed from our gut back into our bloodstream. So, maintaining a balanced microbiome is an often overlooked but essential component of maintaining balanced hormone levels. To maintain a balanced microbiome, it is important to eat a diet rich in fiber and plant phytonutrients.

Another benefit of taking hormones, specifically progesterone, is that it can be beneficial to support a good night's sleep. When we take progesterone, it is metabolized into allopregnanolone. This metabolite can bind to GABA receptors in our brain and help us fall and stay asleep.

When it comes to longevity, hormone replacement therapy (HRT) is one of the lowest-hanging fruits. When it is done in a way that ensures that we have optimal hormone levels and that they are balanced and appropriately metabolized, HRT can have an enormous effect on how we look and feel, not to mention protecting us from many of the diseases of aging.

Reproduction
Accelerated Ovarian Aging Compared to the Rest of the Body

> "Humans are 1 of 5 species on Earth that undergo menopause, including killer whales, short-finned pilot whales, beluga whales, and narwhals."

Ovarian aging refers to the decline of a woman's ovarian reserve, in other words known as the number of oocytes or eggs she has remaining. Females are born with a limited and finite number of eggs, some are released during menstruation, but the majority undergo atresia, when an egg dies and is reabsorbed by the body. This decline of function in ovarian aging occurs roughly 5 times faster than other organ systems in the body, which is referred to as accelerated ovarian aging. At 20 weeks gestation in the womb, a fetal woman has around 6 million eggs, but 1 million or so remain at birth, and only 400,000 for her reproductive years. Eggs come as part of a larger structure in the ovary called a follicle. The follicle contains cells responsible for the production of estrogen. By the age of roughly 54, most women would have completely depleted their ovarian reserve and began menopause despite releasing no more than 500 eggs in their lifetime. In other words, the ovaries have reached the end of their lifespan while the heart is still beating effectively, the brain still operates with only a slight drop in cognition, and muscle mass and lung capacity are at 80% compared to their peaks.

Once menopause begins, there is a sharp drop in estrogen causing a myriad of uncomfortable symptoms including, but not limited to, mood changes, hot flushes, vaginal dryness, low libido, sleep disturbances, and weight gain. At this point a woman is also not able to conceive naturally. Paradoxically, menopause also accelerates the aging of other systems. With low estrogen, the metabolism of the body shifts, which increases the rate of fat deposition in blood vessels increasing the chances of cardiovascular disease. Bones also

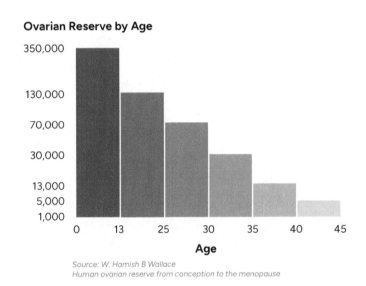

Ovarian Reserve by Age

Source: W. Hamish B Wallace
Human ovarian reserve from conception to the menopause

lose their bone density and become brittle, otherwise known as osteoporotic.

Practicing all longevity habits to maintain optimal metabolic health will also help with fertility and menopause to a degree, although it will not prevent it.

In addition to losing eggs, with age the quality of the eggs that remain also declines, negatively impacting fertility. Ovarian decline is influenced by the starting number of eggs and the speed at which they degrade. As with everything in the body, there is an inherited genetic contribution to one's disposition for ovarian longevity that we cannot control. However, there are some environmental factors that also play a pivotal role. Smoking, poor nutrition, chronic stress, poor sleep hygiene, and being highly under or overweight are associated with a faster decrease in the ovarian reserve and worse outcomes in female fertility.

Good fertility outcomes for women require healthy eggs and a healthy body to host the pregnancy. Lacking this will increase the rate of pregnancy complications. Poor eggs increase the chances of miscarriage and genetic abnormalities in the child. Typically, pregnancy complications are seen to increase from 30 years of age.

Practicing longevity health habits is the best mitigation against environmental influences of ovarian decline, to protect female fertility, and to delay the onset of menopause.

Egg Freezing

While good longevity practices can have a profoundly positive impact on female fertility, the rate of ovarian decline is too great for most women who would like to delay starting their families into their early 30s. Some women also experience premature ovarian insufficiency, an earlier than expected drop in ovarian function and earlier onset of menopause. As a woman's eggs typically are still healthy and present in high numbers during her 20s, the most effective way to preserve fertility is to extract some eggs and freeze them for later use. This means that as a 35-year-old, she can still have a healthy pregnancy using eggs that are frozen at the age of 25.

Despite egg freezing being the most effective, it is currently still impractical despite being practiced since the 1980s. This is because only mature eggs are frozen, and collecting mature eggs has historically been a challenge. In the body, eggs are stored in the ovary in an immature state and mature to be released during menstruation. Only mature eggs are frozen as they freeze and thaw well and can be combined with sperm to make an embryo. Typically, a cocktail of hormones administered over 2 weeks using roughly 24 injections is used to mature the eggs in the body and to stimulate it for release. Once the eggs are ready, they can be extracted by a fertility doctor using ultrasound.

This intense hormone treatment is expensive, requires more of the patient's and clinic's time, and results in a condition called ovarian hyperstimulation syndrome (OHSS). OHSS is caused by these hormone treatments and manifests as uncomfortable side effects in 33% of women with symptoms such as abdominal bloating, abdominal pain, and nausea. These effects are more pronounced in 6% of women, with 1 - 2% requiring urgent hospital treatment. The long-term health effects of these treatments are unknown. Young women who choose to freeze their eggs for voluntary fertility preservation tend to have large ovarian reserves, so they are more likely to experience OHSS as they have a larger amount of follicles able to respond to the hormonal treatment. These are some of the key reasons holding back voluntary egg freezing from common practice.

Gameto's Recent Advances in Fertility Treatments

Improving fertility treatment requires lowering the amount of administered hormones. An alternative protocol called in vitro maturation (IVM) does exist. Essentially, a very small and short regime of hormones is administered (for example, 3 injections over 3 days to extract an immature egg). The egg can be matured in a dish using IVM, which has been practiced since the 2000s but does not deliver sufficiently high pregnancy rates. The reason why IVM is not effective is because it uses static liquid as the nutritive environment for egg maturation. This fails because, in their natural state, eggs mature in an ovary, a living tissue that is able to respond to the needs of the egg and replenish what is needed—unlike the liquid IVM solutions.

Gameto, a biotech company led by CEO and Co-Founder Dr. Dina Radenkovic, is developing treatment solutions to improve women's reproductive health throughout their lives, from egg freezing, infertility, and diseases of the reproductive years to menopause and conditions that occur afterward. The company is revolutionizing the traditional fertility process through innovative therapeutics.

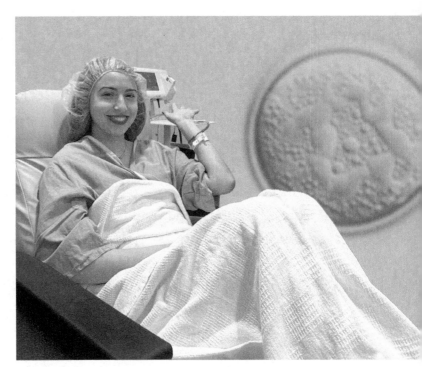

Dina Radenkovic, MD, Co-Founder & CEO, Gameto

Gameto has been developing Fertilo, an IVM product made of engineered ovarian support cells. Fertilo is essentially an ovary in a dish that mimics the natural ovarian environment outside the body. By putting immature eggs in a maturation solution and combining it with Fertilo, the maturation rate of the eggs is roughly 30% higher than using the liquid solution alone. By improving the maturation rate, Fertilo may advance the effectiveness of IVM, allowing women to undergo egg freezing and in vitro fertilization (IVF) procedures with far fewer hormone treatments, meaning lower costs, fewer side effects, and higher safety rates.

These ovarian cells also have other applications. Gameto is using them to engineer Ameno, an implant to produce estrogen a woman is no longer able to produce on her own, allowing the alleviation of menopausal symptoms without the use of hormone replacement therapy. Another application, Deovo, can be used as a platform for drug developers to test the effects of new medicines on the ovaries before releasing drugs to the market. This development has the potential to help unlock many new medicines for young women, who may otherwise miss out due to uncertainties on the effects of the medicine on long-term fertility.

The current trend in research and medical practice that is increasing the focus on female health, in general, and reproductive health, in specific, is reversing the inattention of past decades and is starting to deliver positive results.

Fasting
Intermittent Fasting and Women: A Different Approach

Intermittent fasting has become a widespread trend in recent years, with everyone from celebrities to healthcare professionals singing its praises. And while there is a ton of research suggesting benefits like weight loss, improved blood sugar regulation, and reduced inflammation, we must ask: Is it equally beneficial for women?

Before diving headfirst into intermittent fasting or any proposed longevity practice, we must ask ourselves: *Is this relevant to me as a woman? Are these findings based on studies conducted on women?*

To understand this, let's first acknowledge a key difference between men and women: our fasting insulin levels. Women typically exhibit lower fasting insulin levels, which means our ability to control blood sugar differs significantly from men's.

Now, let's dive deeper into the more nuanced impacts of intermittent fasting on women, particularly the hormonal shifts. Estrogen and progesterone, 2 pivotal female sex hormones, can take a significant hit during prolonged fasting. Intermittent fasting, especially if extended, can interfere with the hormone cycles that women experience monthly. For instance, some women who engage in extended fasts have reported disruptions in their menstrual cycles—sometimes to the point of cessation.

But why does this occur? One could argue that this interruption is nature's ingenious strategy. Consider this: During famines or food shortages, a woman's body might interpret fasting as a signal of scarcity. Such conditions are not ideal for a healthy pregnancy or bringing a baby into a world without food. Hence, by inhibiting ovulation, the body potentially averts pregnancy during times of potential starvation. It's a built-in survival mechanism deeply rooted in our evolutionary biology.

But what are the real-world implications? A decrease in estrogen and progesterone caused by intermittent fasting can trigger a multitude of symptoms, including:

- Changes in the menstrual cycle or skipped periods
- Mood swings
- Night sweats and hot flashes
- Decreased libido
- Sleep disturbances
- Dry skin and hair loss
- Heart palpitations
- Infertility

However, post-menopause, the scenario somewhat shifts. Menopause, typically around the age of 50, marks the cessation of menstrual cycles. Post this phase, estrogen and progesterone levels remain relatively low and consistent. Thus, intermittent fasting might be more effective for post-menopausal women. If post-menopausal women are taking hormone replacement, fasting will not affect the levels of hormone production. Indeed, one study showed that intermittent fasting can be useful for weight loss in post-menopausal women specifically. Yet, caution remains paramount since this was not consistent across studies.

The key thing to remember is that while intermittent fasting might promise a myriad of benefits, as women, we must approach it—and, indeed, all longevity practices—with a tailored lens. We need to question, understand, and then adapt based on what's best for our unique physiology. For example, if you are pregnant, trying to conceive, or have fertility problems, then intermittent fasting should be avoided. The same is true if you are underweight or have a history of an eating disorder. Intermittent fasting can also lead to a loss in muscle mass since your body may try to use muscle for energy. For women, with our lower muscle mass to begin with, this can be problematic. Fasting for extended periods of time can also trigger the stress response and raise cortisol levels. This will add to the breakdown of muscle, bone, and other connective tissue.

Personally, I aim for time-restricted eating. I will stop eating 2 hours before bed and try for 14 to 16 hours of fasting. On days that I am stressed or am doing harder workouts, I will not push that time and settle with an approximately 12-hour eating window.

Toxins

The Unseen Impact of Toxins on Women: My Approach

In our ever-evolving world, we're becoming increasingly aware of the environmental toxins around us and their effects. As women, we are particularly susceptible. There's a reason for this: many toxins find their dwelling in fat tissue, and women, naturally having higher body fat percentages than men, often accumulate more of these harmful agents.

Further exacerbating the issue is our daily routines. On an average day, a woman uses and is exposed to 168 different chemicals from beauty and personal care products. Nail polish, skin creams, shampoos—the list is endless. With societal pressures urging us to look a certain way, we unintentionally increase our chemical exposure in pursuit of these beauty standards.

Some of these toxins contain xenoestrogens, which are external agents that mimic the function of the estrogens our bodies naturally produce. Not naturally synthesized by our body, they are pervasive in items like plastics, tap water, canned food, and even laundry products. Binding to estrogen receptors, they produce effects similar to natural estrogens, leading to a condition termed "estrogen dominance." Symptoms like breast swelling and pain often aren't just an effect of our body's hormones but are influenced by these external intruders.

To combat these invisible threats, I've taken a proactive approach. I choose personal care products that are organic and have minimal additives. I stay away from parabens, phthalates, and acrylamides, but there are so many more sources of toxins. SafeCosmetics.org/Chemicals lists many of these harmful compounds.

Recognizing that toxins aren't limited to beauty products, I prioritize organic food. By doing so, I aim to minimize the potential harm from dietary sources containing herbicides and pesticides.

Our understanding of the health impacts from toxins in our environment continues to expand. In medical school, it was traditionally taught that men rarely faced bone density loss until advanced age. However, now we witness it in men as young as 30 and even more prominently in women. While the exact causes remain elusive, there's growing suspicion that toxins are a significant player.

The truth is that toxins are ubiquitous in the world we live in. But my mantra is simple: Control what's within your grasp and release undue stress over the rest. We can't eliminate every toxin, but by being aware and making informed choices, we can make a significant difference in our health and well-being.

Stress
Dealing With Stress and Anxiety as a Woman

It's a broadly acknowledged reality: anxiety and stress are more prevalent in women than men. Think about the various roles women wear—caregivers, mothers, daughters caring for aging parents, stewards of the home, professionals in the workforce—the list is extensive. The sheer volume of responsibilities thrust upon us can often feel overwhelming.

And the stress it creates infiltrates every inch of our being. From our mental faculties to our very cells, no part remains untouched. It calls for self-care, not as a luxury but as a necessity to remain robust and thriving. However, the implications of stress stretch further than our immediate sensations of unease. Chronic stress has insidious companions: exhaustion, anxiety, panic, and anger. Left unchecked, these can spiral into burnout and even a complete breakdown.

Venturing deeper, the ripples of stress resonate within our endocrine system, particularly our hormones. Have you heard of "progesterone steal"? Stress cunningly diverts our hormone metabolism, prioritizing the production of cortisol over our crucial sex hormones.

But before we brand stress as the unequivocal adversary, let's pause. Stress, in its optimal amounts, is a valuable ally. It's the sweet spot where performance thrives. Too little, and we lack the drive; too much, and we risk derailment.

Having grappled with stress throughout my life, I've endeavored not to internalize external pressures. I've worked hard in my life not to take things personally, and while I'm not always successful, I've found this has helped me a lot.

I also use binaural beats. It essentially connects both halves of your brain by using a slightly different auditory signal in each ear. When you listen to it in stereo, your brain is trying to make sense of what's going on, and as a result, it connects both halves. You can actually entrain your brainwaves into different alpha, delta, and theta brainwave patterns.

Additionally, being outside is a hugely helpful stress reliever for me. I love walking in nature. Finally, and perhaps most importantly, remember to cultivate and maintain your key relationships—social support is critical for managing stress and anxiety.

It is important to do what we can to optimize our health and longevity by following all these practices. However, we are not always going to be perfect. Sometimes, what we know will benefit us may not be enjoyable. For example, I really don't like being cold. Cold plunges may have a wonderful hormetic effect on longevity, but I choose not to do them very often because even just the thought of an ice-cold shower or bath causes me stress, and I can feel my whole body tighten.

So, just like with toxins, do what you can, control what you can, and then don't worry about the rest since the stress of worrying about doing everything just right is detrimental in and of itself.

Exercise
Should Women Exercise Differently than Men?

Although there is an almost universal understanding that both men and women reap tremendous benefits from exercise, there has been an unwritten code that women should opt for cardio, yoga, and fitness classes while men should lift weights, play competitive sports, and do high-intensity training. And while we now understand the importance of muscle mass in health and longevity for both men and women, only 17% of women regularly lift weights while outnumbering men in yoga and group fitness classes by 5:1.

Does this difference in the type of exercise that women and men engage in make physiological sense, or is it a result of societal conditioning? While we may want to blame stereotypes, there are similarities and differences in how men and women respond to exercise. While men inherently have more muscle mass and larger muscle fibers compared to women, when body weight is considered, women with proper training can develop equal strength ratios. Women also tend to build lower body muscle mass more quickly, while men can increase upper body muscle more easily. During weight training, women can take shorter rest periods between sets since they can recover faster. Women tend to burn more sugar during rest but can burn fat more efficiently during exercise, especially weight training and high-intensity training.

When refueling after exercise, women may not need the carbohydrate refueling and do better with a balanced post-workout meal. As mentioned above, in intermittent fasting, men respond well to calorie deficits or high intensity for fat loss, while women are more likely to experience a stress response and cortisol release, resulting in fat storage with intense training or significant calorie deficits.

I try to make exercise a priority. I do Zone 2 training as my base. This is a fast walk for me and allows me to get outside, experience nature, and catch up on podcasts or Audible books. I add body weight training and kettlebells 2 - 3 times a week. As part of my kettlebell routine, I try to achieve short, high-intensity heart rate bursts of 1 - 2 minutes to push my VO2 max capacity. I also make sure to incorporate appropriate recovery and stretching along with my favorite post-workout Ka'Chava shake. While yoga may be a female stereotype, it still provides significant benefits, and I try to incorporate it daily for both flexibility and stability.

In addition, I try to add movement to my regular routine. I use a standing desk and often do standing tree pose on one leg during my meetings, in addition to 20 squats after every meeting. This keeps oxygen flowing to my brain and helps to stabilize my blood sugar. Another trick I often do is whole-body static muscle contractions during meetings, which can be done without anyone noticing and helps to build strength.

Sleep

Do Women Really Need More Sleep than Men?

The importance of sleep for longevity has been well outlined in the previous chapters, but is there a gender difference when it comes to how much sleep we need? It turns out that, on average, women need slightly more sleep than men, to the tune of 20 minutes, and they also tend to get more deep sleep. There are also sex differences in circadian rhythm, where women's circadian rhythms tend to shift earlier than men's, which means you might feel sleepier in the evening and wake up earlier in the morning.

Hormones can also play a role in sleep, and often, women report better sleep in the first half of their cycle when estrogen predominates. Hormones can also affect body temperature, which can then have an impact on sleep. Using a cooling sleep mattress that can be adjusted based on monthly cycles is an excellent way to compensate for this.

Supplements & Medications
What Do I Take? It Depends.

When people ask me what supplements I take, I always say, "It depends." I don't take the same supplements every day. I typically buy a range of supplements wholesale, keep them at home, and then choose the supplements to take for a given week based on how I feel.

I recently took an inventory of all the supplements I have in my cupboard, and I've included a summary of them below. Note: I've tried to group these into categories, but many of these supplements will overlap across categories. I also try to use products that contain many ingredients in one capsule to limit the number of capsules I take.

Remember that the dosing of supplements should be modified for women and is unique to you, your physiology, and desired outcomes. Based on our smaller body size and unique metabolism, the standard dosing that has been determined for men may not be applicable to us, and we often need lower doses. Ultimately, dosing and frequency will be determined between you and your physician.

Gut & Microbiome Support

- **Digestive Enzyme With Food (typically with each large meal)**: Our ability to make stomach acid decreases as we get older. Stress also decreases our ability to make stomach acid, so I take a digestive enzyme to ensure that I get all the benefits of the food I eat and can fully digest and absorb all of the nutrients.

- **Butyrate**: Butyrate is a short-chain fatty acid made from fiber by the microbes in our gut. It keeps the lining of our GI tract healthy and prevents leaky gut. By taking butyrate, I can support my gut lining and create an environment for the good microbes in my gut to thrive.

- **TUDCA**: Tauroursodeoxycholic Acid or TUDCA is a bile acid derivative that occurs naturally in the body and is made by microbes when they metabolize the bile acids that are released into our intestines by our liver. TUDCA has been shown to support brain function, liver, kidney, eye, mitochondria and cellular health, insulin sensitivity, gut microbiome balance, and bile flow, which help digestion of fats.

- **Fiber**: I take a variety of different fiber supplements. Fiber is one of the most important things to maintain a healthy microbiome. It acts as a fuel for the beneficial microbes. Just like with our food, it is important to get a variety of different fibers, so I will rotate a number of different supplements with different types of fiber. I usually add it to a shake or sprinkle on my food.

- **N-Acetyl-glucosamine (NAG)**: Provides building blocks for the intestinal glycocalyx, which is the inside coating of the gut that protects us from leaky gut. NAG has also been shown to increase the elasticity of tissues surrounding blood vessels and support immune health.

Cardiovascular

- **Nattokinase**: Nattokinase is a very safe blood thinner that prevents clotting and can be helpful if you travel a lot or do a lot of sitting to prevent blood clot formation.

- **Arterosil**: Arterosil is a glycocalyx regenerating compound and has been shown to build and maintain the endothelial glycocalyx. This is the inner coating of all our blood vessels. When this structure breaks down, it is the first step in atherosclerosis and damage to our vessel's walls.

- **Vascanox**: Vascanox increases the production of nitric oxide, which is needed to dilate our blood vessels. This can maintain healthy blood vessels and blood pressure.

- **Omega-3 Fatty Acids**: Omega 3 fatty acids are a component of our cell membranes. They are precursors to the anti-inflammatory molecules of our immune system. The fatty acids we take need to be balanced. That is, we need the right ratios of omega 3 to omega 6 as well as saturated fatty acids. Most of us do not get enough omega 3. It benefits our brain and heart and reduces overall inflammation.

Brain Health

- **Prodrome Neuro and Gila Plasmalogens**: These are important components of our cell's membranes, especially in our brain. As we get older, our levels of plasmalogens decrease. Low plasmalogen levels are associated with poor cognitive function and dementia.

- **Omega-3 Fatty Acids**: As above, our neurons need omega 3 fatty acids to be healthy.

- **Phosphatidylcholine (PC)**: Phosphatidylcholine makes up most of our cell membranes. Choline is also used to make acetylcholine, which is a critical neurotransmitter in our brains and is predominantly used by our vagus nerve. So, PC can help with mood, memory, stress, and even muscle control.

- **Ketone Esters (e.g., Cognitive Switch from Juvenescence)**: Ketones are amazing fuel for our brain. We make ketones when we fast or follow a ketogenic diet. We can take them as a supplement, and they can protect our brain and enhance cognitive function. I take them whenever I need a brain boost.

Cellular / Mitochondrial Support

- **Coenzyme Q10**: CoQ10 is essential for energy production in the mitochondria. It is also a powerful antioxidant.

- **Curcumin**: Curcumin is found in turmeric and has an enormous number of beneficial effects, most notably as an anti-inflammatory substance.

- **Multivitamins**: I take a multivitamin to supply my basic vitamin and mineral needs. I use one in food form with added greens and other phytonutrients, including resveratrol.

- **Acetyl-L-Carnitine**: Carnitine is needed to shuttle fatty acids into the mitochondria, the Acetyl form can get into the brain. It helps with energy production and blood sugar regulation.

Stress & Sleep

- **Phyto ADR Adaptogens**: Adaptogens are a class of herbs that help the body adapt to physical, chemical, or biological stressors. They have been used in traditional Chinese and Ayurvedic medicine for centuries. When I am under stress, these can really be helpful. I always make sure they contain ashwagandha, rhodiola, and ginseng.

- **Phosphatidylserine (PS)**: PS is part of our cell membranes. It can help manage the stress response as well as improve memory and cognitive function. It is great to help sleep on those stressful days.

- **Magnesium Glycinate**: Magnesium is essential for more than 300 biochemical reactions. We tend to use up magnesium when we are under stress. If we ever get tight muscles or constipation, it is often a sign of a need for magnesium. I will adjust my dose of magnesium based on the kind of day I have had.

- **Glycine**: Glycine is an amino acid that makes up the majority of collagen. It is also a precursor to glutathione and supports detoxification pathways in the liver. Glycine also acts as an inhibitory neurotransmitter in the brain, promoting relaxation and sleep.

- **Melatonin**: Melatonin is produced by our pineal gland and regulates our sleep/wake cycle. It helps to set and keep our circadian rhythms on track. It is also an amazing antioxidant and supports eye, GI, heart, and brain health. It also protects mitochondria and has anti-cancer effects.

Toxins

- **N-Acetyl Cysteine (NAC)/Glutathione**: Glutathione is our major detoxifier and antioxidant, in our toxic world, it is critical to maintain our levels. NAC is the rate-limiting step to making glutathione, so I always make sure I get enough to support my glutathione production.

Longevity

- **Glucosamine**: Glucosamine sulfate has been shown in large human studies to be correlated with increased lifespan. It is associated with a reduced risk of cardiovascular disease and a lower incidence of diabetes. It supports the production of mitochondria and reduces inflammaging.

- **Carnosine**: Carnosine is a dipeptide found in brain and muscle tissue. It protects against glycation and can counteract age-related cellular damage.

- **Low-dose Lithium**: Low-dose lithium has been linked to longer lifespan in epidemiological studies and enhances the health of neurons.
- **Taurine**: Taurine is an amino acid found abundantly in the brain, retina, heart, and platelets. It supports cardiovascular health, and recent studies show it can mitigate some age-related declines in organ function.
- **TruNiagin and Niacin**: TruNiagin is a form of NR that can increase NAD+ levels, and niacin also supports NAD+ levels as well as healthy lipid levels.
- **Quercetin**: A flavonoid found in many fruits and vegetables, Quercetin has been studied as a senolytic. It also has strong antioxidant and anti-inflammatory effects and can protect against cellular damage.
- **Spermidine**: Spermidine is a natural polyamine found in certain foods and is made by our microbiome from fermentable fibers. It is known to induce autophagy and may also support cardiovascular health, reduce inflammation, and extend lifespan in animal models.
- **Fisetin**: Fisetin is a naturally occurring flavonoid found in various fruits and vegetables such as strawberries and apples. It has been investigated for its potential to promote longevity by acting as an antioxidant and anti-inflammatory, and it may also be a powerful senolytic.
- **Pterostilbene**: A natural compound found in foods like blueberries and grapes. It has been studied for its potential benefits in promoting longevity due to its ability to protect cells from damage with its antioxidant and anti-inflammatory potential.
- **Alpha-Ketoglutarate (AKG):** A compound involved in the Krebs cycle, a critical metabolic pathway in the body needed to make energy. AKG supplementation may have benefits in promoting longevity by influencing mitochondrial function and cellular energy production.

Muscle & Skin Health

- **Collagen**: Protein to promote skin health.
- **Whey Protein**: Good, easily digestible source of protein to help maintain my muscle mass.
- **HMB**: Beta-hydroxy beta-methylbutyrate is a metabolite of the amino acid leucine. It has been studied for its potential to counteract sarcopenia by promoting muscle protein synthesis and reducing muscle protein breakdown to help preserve muscle mass and strength.

I hope these longevity practices are helpful to my fellow women out there.

Here's to your health and longevity!

Appendix A:
Blue Zone Wisdom

"I believe that aging is a disease. I believe it is treatable. I believe we can treat it within our lifetimes. And in doing so, I believe, everything we know about human health will be fundamentally changed."

—David Sinclair, PhD

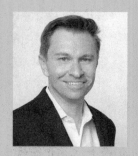

The Blue Zones are regions of the world where people are known to live longer, healthier lives compared to the rest of the population. These areas have been identified through research conducted by the Blue Zones Project. Based on research by Dan Buettner, a National Geographic Fellow and *New York Times* bestselling author, 5 cultures of the world—or blue zones—were identified with the highest concentration of people living to be 100 years or older.

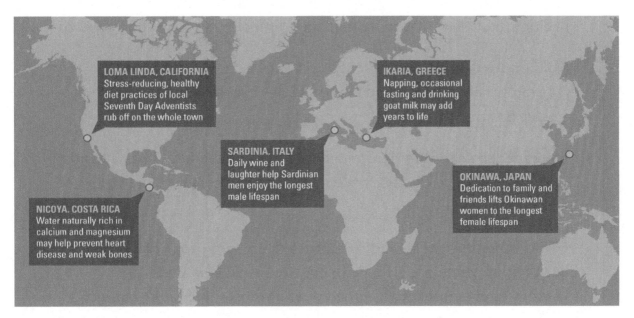

Blue Zone Map shows where today's centenarians are concentrated
https://www.webmd.com/healthy-aging/ss/slideshow-longer-life-secrets

18 "Blue Zone" Secrets for a Longer Life

Following are 18 identified hallmarks of centenarians living in Blue Zones.
How many are you following?

1. **Protect Your DNA**: Safeguard your genetic material by avoiding exposure to harmful toxins and adopting a healthy lifestyle. Use sunscreen and avoid too much sun exposure. Preventing DNA damage promotes overall longevity.

2. **Play to Win**: Approach life with a positive and competitive mindset, setting goals and challenges for yourself. This is important because it keeps your mind engaged, fosters resilience, and adds purpose to your existence.

3. **Make Friends/Community**: Cultivate meaningful relationships and engage with your community regularly. This fosters a support system that provides emotional well-being and a sense of belonging, which are essential for a long, fulfilling life.

4. **Choose Friends Wisely**: Surround yourself with people who uplift and support you in your journey. Your social circle profoundly influences your habits, attitudes, and outlook, impacting your overall health and longevity.

5. **Quit Smoking**: Break free from the grip of tobacco to protect your respiratory health and reduce the risk of life-threatening diseases. If you smoke, quit now.

6. **Embrace the Art of the Nap**: Incorporate short, restorative naps into your routine to recharge your body and mind. Napping enhances productivity and mental clarity.

7. **Follow a Mediterranean Diet**: Prioritize a diet rich in vegetables, whole grains, healthy fats, and fish. The Mediterranean diet is associated with lower rates of chronic diseases and promotes heart health, increasing your chances of longevity.

8. **Eat Like an Okinawan**: Model your eating habits after the Okinawan diet, emphasizing plant-based foods and lean protein sources. This dietary choice is linked to exceptional longevity and vitality.

9. **Get Hitched**: Cultivate a loving, committed relationship or marriage. Married individuals, on average, live longer, with a mortality rate about 15% lower than unmarried individuals.

10. **Lose Weight**: Achieve and maintain a healthy weight through balanced eating and regular exercise. Weight management is essential for preventing chronic diseases and improving overall well-being.

11. **Keep Moving**: Stay physically active through daily exercise and movement. Regular activity boosts circulation and maintains muscle and bone health, enhancing longevity.

12. **Drink in Moderation**: Consume alcohol in moderation to protect your liver and overall health. Reduced alcohol promotes longevity.

13. **Get Spiritual**: Cultivate a sense of spirituality or purpose that gives your life meaning and direction. Spiritual practices can reduce stress and enhance mental and emotional well-being.

14. **Forgive**: Let go of grudges and practice forgiveness to reduce emotional stress and foster healthier relationships. Forgiveness enables mental and emotional longevity.

15. **Use Safety Gear**: Prioritize safety in your activities by wearing appropriate gear (seat belts, ski helmet) and taking precautions. This helps prevent accidents and injuries that can disrupt a long and healthy life.

16. **Make Sleep a Priority**: Prioritize quality sleep by maintaining a consistent sleep schedule and creating a restful environment. Good sleep habits are fundamental for physical and mental rejuvenation.

17. **Manage Stress**: Implement stress-reduction techniques such as meditation, deep breathing, or mindfulness. Effective stress management is crucial for both mental and physical health and longevity.

18. **Keep a Sense of Purpose**: Cultivate a clear sense of purpose in life, whether through work, hobbies, or community involvement. A sense of purpose enhances motivation and resilience, contributing to a fulfilling and longer life.

Appendix B: Recommended Reading

"Knowledge is the antidote to fear."

—Ralph Waldo Emerson

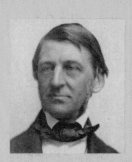

Here are my top 10 reading recommendations if you care to dive in deeper. Note: these are not provided in any particular order; all are brilliant.

Life Force: How New Breakthroughs in Precision Medicine Can Transform the Quality of Your Life & Those You Love,
by Tony Robbins, Peter H. Diamandis, MD, and Robert Hariri, MD, PhD (2022)

Lifespan: Why We Age—and Why We Don't Have To,
by David Sinclair, PhD (2019)

Outlive: The Science and Art of Longevity,
by Peter Attia, MD (2022)

Why We Sleep: Unlocking the Power of Sleep and Dreams,
by Matthew Walker, PhD (2017)

The Science and Technology of Growing Young: An Insider's Guide to the Breakthroughs that Will Dramatically Extend Our Lifespan . . . and What You Can Do Right Now,
by Sergey Young (2021)

Young Forever: Live Longer, Healthier, and Happier Using the Latest Science,
by Mark Hyman, MD (2022)

The Kaufmann Protocol: Why We Age and How to Stop It,
by Sandra Kaufmann, MD (2018)

Fantastic Voyage: Live Long Enough to Live Forever,
by Ray Kurzweil (2004)

Ageless: The New Science of Getting Older Without Getting Old,
by Andrew Steele, PhD (2021)

Ending Aging: The Rejuvenation Breakthroughs That Could Reverse Human Aging in Our Lifetime,
by Aubrey de Grey, PhD (2008)

Appendix C:
Product Recommendations

"The best way to predict the future is to create it yourself."

—Peter H. Diamandis, MD

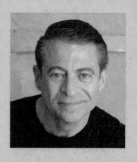

Here's a list of products that I personally use and that have been mentioned throughout this book.

Athletic Greens AG1 – https://diamandis.net/ag1

Nutri11 by Dr. Guillermo R. Navarrete – https://diamandis.net/Nutri11

MUD\WTR: A Coffee Alternative – https://diamandis.net/mud

ProLon Fasting Mimicking Diet (FMD) – https://diamandis.net/prolonfast

Levels Health Continuous Glucose Monitor – https://diamandis.net/levels

FreeStyle LibreLink – https://diamandis.net/FreeStyle

Oura Ring – https://diamandis.net/oura

Katalyst Electrical Muscle Stimulation Suit – http://diamandis.net/katalyst

Tonal – https://diamandis.net/tonal

InBody H20N Smart Full Body Composition Analyzer – https://diamandis.net/inbody

Manta Sleep Mask – https://diamandis.net/manta

Audible – https://diamandis.net/audible

Eight Sleep Cooling Mattress Pad – https://diamandis.net/eightsleep

Lifeforce Products: – https://diamandis.net/lifeforce
- Peak Rest
- Peak Rise
- Peak Healthspan
- Peak NMN

Fountain Life Apex Membership – https://diamandis.net/fountainlife

OneSkin's OS-1 – https://diamandis.net/oneskin

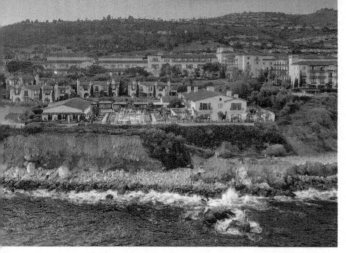

The Annual Summit is held at the beautiful Terranea Resort in Los Angeles, CA

abundance 360
By Singularity University

How do you keep up with exponential change?

We will experience more change this coming decade than we have in the entire past century.

Converging exponential technologies like AI, Robotics, AR/VR, Quantum, and Biotech are disrupting and reinventing every industry and business model.

How do you surf this tsunami of change, survive, and thrive?

The answer lies in your access to **Knowledge** and **Community**.

Knowledge about the breakthroughs expected over the next two to three years.

This Knowledge comes from an incredible Faculty curated by Peter H. Diamandis, MD, at his private leadership summit held each March called ***Abundance360***.

Every year, Peter gathers Faculty who are industry disruptors and changemakers. Picture yourself learning from visionaries and having conversations with leaders such as **Cathie Wood**, **Palmer Luckey**, **Jacqueline Novogratz**, **Sam Altman**, **Marc Benioff**, **Tony Robbins**, **Eric Schmidt**, **Ray Kurzweil**, **Andrew Yang**, **Emad Mostaque**, **will.i.am**, **Sal Khan**, **Arianna Huffington**, **Salim Ismail**, **Andrew Ng**, and **Martine Rothblatt** (just to name a handful over the past few years).

Even more important than Knowledge is **Community**.

A Community that understands your challenges and inspires you to pursue your Massive Transformative Purpose (MTP) and Moonshot(s).

Community is core to Abundance360. Our members are hand-selected and carefully cultivated—fellow entrepreneurs, investors, business owners, and CEOs running businesses valued from $10M to $10B.

Abundance360 is a global community of entrepreneurs, CEOs & investors changing the world

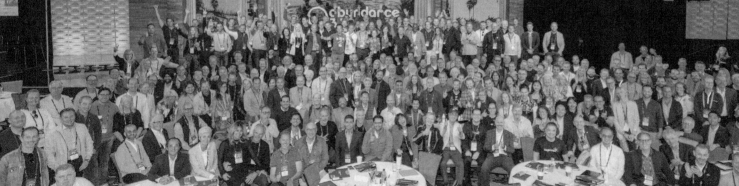

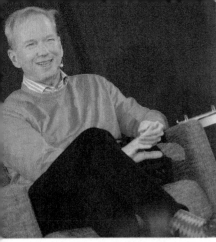

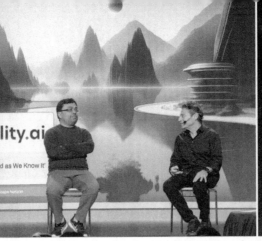

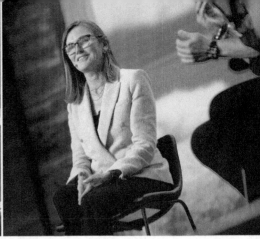

Eric Schmidt, Co-Founder, Schmidt Futures & Former CEO, Google

Peter speaks with Emad Mostaque, Founder & CEO, Stability.ai

Cathie Wood, Founder, CEO, CIO, ARKInvest

Abundance360 members believe that "The day before something is truly a breakthrough, it's a crazy idea." They also believe that "We are living during the most extraordinary time ever in human history!"

Having the right Knowledge and Community can be the difference between thriving in your business—or getting disrupted and crushed by the tsunami of change.

This is the essence of Abundance360: Singularity University's highest-level leadership program that includes an annual 3 ½ day Summit, hands-on quarterly Workshops, regular Masterminds, one-on-one member matching, and a vibrant, close-knit Community with an uncompromising Mission.

> **"We're here to shape your mindset, fuel your ambitions with cutting-edge technologies, accelerate your wealth, and amplify your global impact."**

Admission to Abundance360 is only through invitation or referrals from current members. If you're interested in joining our Community, visit **Abundance360.com** to learn more.

> **"I'm in the process of selling my business for much more and I've made many millions due to what I've learned at A360."**
> *- Jeff Peoples, CEO, Structural Macrotrend Fund LP*

> **"I have grown my company 10x, thanks to A360. We're in hyper scale mode."**
> *- Blake Miller, CEO, Homebase.ai*

> **"A360 is among the most valuable and transformative decisions I've ever made."**
> *- David Erickson, Co-Founder, Promise Hub*

Members explore VR & other exponential tech

Your community shapes what you do

Ameca, one of the world's leading humanoid robots

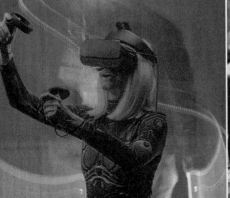

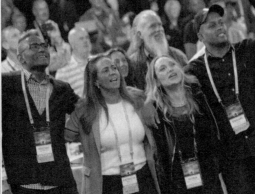

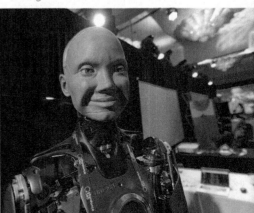

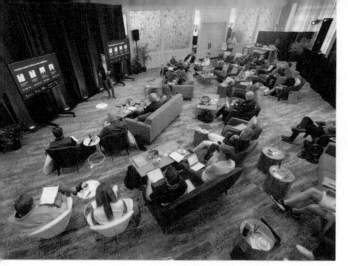

Learn from the top scientists & entrepreneurs in longevity/biotech

ABUNDANCE
PLATINUM

By Singularity University

Interested in the latest biotech breakthroughs?

How AI is designing new medications? How epigenetic reprogramming is reversing aging, or how to regrow human organs?

Perhaps you're interested in accessing the top longevity-related investment opportunities? Or finding breakthrough treatments for a loved one?

If yes, then consider joining Peter H. Diamandis, MD, on his annual **Abundance Platinum Longevity Trip**.

Every year, Peter runs two VIP "Abundance Platinum Longevity Trips," which are 5-Day/5-Star deep dives into the cutting-edge world of biotech/longevity and age reversal.

On odd years (2019, 2021, 2023…), the trip takes place in the Northeast of the U.S. in Boston, Cambridge, New Hampshire, and New York City. On even years (2020, 2022, 2024…), the trip takes place on the west coast of the U.S. in San Francisco/Bay Area and San Diego.

Each Trip is capped at 40 participants every September and 40 participants every October. This keeps the group size small and intimate, ensuring that all participants have full access to all elements of the experience.

Members visit the best of the longevity/biotech ecosystems on both coasts (Boston/Cambridge pictured here)

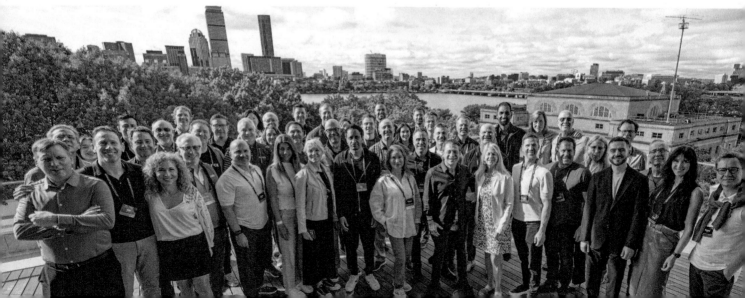